Get Through

FRCR Part 1: MCQs and Mock Examination

To our families and our teachers

Get Through
FRCR Part 1: MCQs and Mock Examination

Damian Tolan MBChB MRCP(UK)
Specialist Registrar in Diagnostic Radiology, Leeds

Rachel Hyland MBChB
Specialist Registrar in Diagnostic Radiology, Leeds

Christopher Taylor BSc
Head of Radiological Physics, Radiation Protection Adviser and Head of Leeds FRCR Physics Teaching Programme, Leeds Teaching Hospitals Trust

Arnold Cowen BSc
Senior Lecturer in Medical Physics, University of Leeds

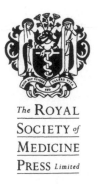

The ROYAL
SOCIETY of
MEDICINE
PRESS Limited

© 2004 Royal Society of Medicine Press Ltd

Published by the Royal Society of Medicine Press Ltd
1 Wimpole Street, London W1G 0AE, UK
Tel: +44 (0)20 7290 2921
Fax: +44 (0)20 7290 2929
E-mail: publishing@rsm.ac.uk
Website: www.rsmpress.co.uk

British Library Cataloguing in Publication Data
A catalogue record for this book is available from the British Library

ISBN 1-85315-578-0

Distribution in Europe and Rest of World:

Marston Book Services Ltd
PO Box 269
Abingdon
Oxon OX14 4YN, UK
Tel: +44 (0)1235 465500
Fax: +44 (0)1235 465555

Distribution in the USA and Canada:

Royal Society of Medicine Press Ltd
c/o Jamco Distribution Inc
1401 Lakeway Drive
Lewisville, TX 75057, USA
Tel: +1 800 538 1287
Fax: +1 972 353 1303
E-mail: jamco@majors.com

Distribution in Australia and New Zealand:

Elsevier Australia
30–52 Smidmore Street
Marrickville NSW 2204, Australia
Tel: + 61 2 9517 8999
Fax: + 61 2 9517 2249
E-mail: service@elsevier.com.au

Phototypeset by Phoenix Photosetting, Chatham, Kent
Printed in the UK by Bell & Bain, Glasgow

Contents

Foreword

As radiologists we rely heavily on the "Aunt Minnie" pattern recognition approach to interpret our images. Short-cutting a careful visual analysis in this way works well most of the time, but after over 30 years in clinical radiology I still see – every week – new or unfamiliar appearances which fit no clear pattern but which require explanation. In these circumstances, the question we need to ask is not "what is it?" but rather "what has happened to produce these appearances?" In part, this is an exploration of how the pathology or pathophysiology in the patient has become manifest in the image – we have to back-project the substance from the shadow. However, the other critical element to our visual analysis requires us to understand the technical aspects of image acquisition and display, and for this reason it is important for radiologists to have a firm understanding of the science and technology involved in image production.

The last four decades have seen a dramatic expansion in the range of clinical imaging techniques and the role of the radiologist has evolved equally rapidly. Fortunately, the basic science remains the same as it always was. In reading through this book I was reassured to find that in an increasingly ephemeral world, protons and electrons continue to be unimpressed by politics and post-modernism. Once you have digested this book, its contents will provide you with long-term sustenance.

The authors are amongst the first students and teachers to experience the revised syllabus and examination for Part 1 of the FRCR in December 2002. In a format which is clear and concise they have covered the radiation physics relevant to imaging - including x-radiography, computed tomography and radionuclide imaging - also those aspects of radiation protection which are relevant to clinical applications, and all the accompanying legislation. This volume will be invaluable not only to candidates for the FRCR part 1, but as a continuing source of reference to radiologists at a later stage of their training and experience. The authors are to be congratulated on this most valuable contribution.

Philip JA Robinson
Professor of Clinical Radiology
St James's University Hospital
Leeds

Abbreviations

ARSAC	administration of radioactive substances advisory committee
Bq	becquerel (disintegrations per second)
c	speed of light ($3 \times 10^8 \text{ms}^{-1}$)
C	coulomb
CTDI	Computed tomography dose index
DAP	dose area product (Gy cm^2, cGy cm^2)
DRL	diagnostic reference level
eV	electron volts ($1 \text{ eV} = 1.6 \times 10^{-19}$ joules); subdivisions are keV and MeV
f	frequency
FFD	focus film distance
Gy	gray – a unit of absorbed dose, and of kerma; subdivisions are mGy and µGy
mGy cm	milligray-centimetres, a unit of dose–length product
h	Planck's constant (6.626×10^{-34} Js)
HVL	half value layer
HSE	Health and Safety Executive
IRR 1999	Ionising Radiations Regulations 1999
IRMER	Ionising Radiation (Medical Exposure) Regulations 2000
kV	kilovolt
kVp	peak electrical potential across an x-ray tube, in kilovolts
kW	kilowatt
LAC	linear attenuation coefficient
lp/mm	line pairs per millimetre
mA	milliamperes (tube current)
mAs	milliampere-seconds
MBq/mg	megabecquerel per milligram, a unit of specific activity
MTF	modulation transfer function
rad	radiation absorbed dose (a non-SI unit of absorbed dose or kerma)
SI	Système Internationale
Sv	sievert – a unit of effective dose and equivalent dose; subdivisions are mSv and µSv
TLD	thermoluminescent dose meter
Z	atomic number
λ	wavelength

The text uses standard chemical symbols, e.g. Tc (technetium) and CsI (caesium iodide). Nuclides have been written with either the name or symbol of the element followed by its atomic mass number, e.g. technetium-99 or Tc-99.

Introduction

Radiology is the most competitive and rapidly expanding specialty in medicine. Advances in technology and new legislation have driven a change in the examination structure by the Royal College of Radiologists. The new part 1 FRCR examination was introduced in December 2002 and covers basic physics and radiation safety, with the aim that candidates move into practical specialist training earlier in their training. The exam is held three times a year at five UK centres and in Dublin, Singapore and Hong Kong. No minimum period of clinical experience or clinical radiology training is needed to enter the examination, nor is attendance on a physics course compulsory. This means that for the first time it is open to non-radiology trainees who are hoping to enter specialist training in the future.

We intended to provide accurate questions representative in style and content of the new exam, including more difficult topics, and to help students learn essential facts and direct further reading in areas of weakness. Half of the new syllabus and questions in the two first examinations were dedicated to legislation (IRR 1999, IRMER 2000), a topic not covered in currently available textbooks, but included and emphasised in our book.

The need to set questions with true or false answers has posed us a number of problems, as it surely must for the FRCR examiners. We have tried as far as possible to make our questions unambiguous, without trivialising them, but there may be some room for discussion of some of the answers. Please bear in mind that things change, and that some of our information will only be true at the time of writing. Hopefully, the physics will not change, and the recently enacted legislation will be around for a while.

We hope that the layout of our book will allow candidates to use the questions for revision and to test examination technique. A separate mock examination has been provided at the end of the book for this purpose. We have specifically tried to provide clear, detailed explanations in answer to our questions and hope that they clarify difficult parts of the syllabus. This book should also be of use to radiographers in undergraduate and postgraduate training programmes for revision, and radiography and medical physics lecturers in writing questions for their courses.

Finally, we wish you good luck and every success in the exam!

I. Fundamental properties of matter, radiation and radioactive decay

1.1 **Concerning electromagnetic radiation:**

a. Unattenuated radiation travels in straight lines.
b. The inverse square law applies equally to both extended and point sources of radiation.
c. The inverse square law applies to all types of high energy electromagnetic radiation.
d. It is composed of particles and waves.
e. It comprises electric and magnetic fields oscillating perpendicular to each other and to the direction of propagation.

1.2 **Regarding electromagnetic radiation:**

a. The frequency of the electromagnetic radiation is directly proportional to the photon energy.
b. The energy of a photon of electromagnetic radiation is typically expressed in joules.
c. The speed of a photon increases with the energy of the beam.
d. The speed of electromagnetic radiation is independent of the medium through which it travels.
e. Gamma and x-ray photons differ from each other in frequency and wavelength.

1.3 **The following examples are types of electromagnetic radiation:**

a. Light.
b. Microwaves.
c. Sound waves.
d. Gamma rays.
e. Beta radiation.

1.4 **All forms of ionising radiation:**

a. Are used in diagnostic medical imaging.
b. Are attenuated exponentially in matter.
c. Can cause cell damage.
d. Obey the inverse square law.
e. May cause heating.

3

1.5 **Regarding the nucleus:**

a. The atomic mass number is the number of protons in an atom.
b. The atomic number defines the element.
c. A nucleus may only exist at only one energy level.
d. Neutrons and protons are loosely associated within the nucleus.
e. A radionuclide is a nuclide whose atoms are unstable.

1.6 **Nuclides:**

a. Are components of the nucleus.
b. Are radioactive.
c. Of the same element with different atomic masses are called isotopes.
d. Are defined by their atomic mass number only.
e. Are fully defined by their atomic mass number and atomic number.

1.7 **Concerning atoms:**

a. The numbers of protons and neutrons are equal in a stable nucleus.
b. In a tungsten atom, transitions from L shells are more likely than from K shells.
c. Electron binding energy is the energy required to promote an electron to a higher energy orbital shell.
d. Using the helium atom as an example, the K shell contains four electrons.
e. Positrons and electrons are of equal mass.

1.8 **Regarding electron orbital shells:**

a. Electrons exist in a continuous spectrum of energy levels around the nucleus.
b. The binding energy of the K shell is always greater than that of the other shells.
c. The valence shell is the source of characteristic radiation.
d. Atomic number has no influence on the K shell binding energy.
e. Each shell may only contain a set maximum number of electrons.

1.9 **Concerning electrons traversing an x-ray tube during a radiographic exposure:**

a. They travel from anode to cathode.
b. They ultimately dissipate most of their kinetic energy as heat.
c. They are deflected by electric fields.
d. The electron volt is a quantity only used to measure electron energy.
e. They are unaffected by a loss of the vacuum seal in the tube.

1.10 There is no change in the atomic number of an element after the following processes:

a. Isomeric transition.
b. K shell capture.
c. Internal conversion.
d. Positron emission.
e. Chemical shift.

1.11 Radioactive decay may be directly accompanied by the following types of emission:

a. Positron emission.
b. Gamma rays.
c. Alpha particles.
d. Bremsstrahlung.
e. Characteristic x-radiation.

1.12 All of the isotopes of an element:

a. Have different atomic numbers.
b. Have different atomic masses.
c. Occupy the same position in the periodic table.
d. Decay by emitting ionising radiation.
e. If they are gamma emitters, they will emit the same frequency of radiation.

1.13 With radioactive decay:

a. Metastable nuclides tend to release gamma radiation to reach a stable ground state.
b. Alpha emission reduces the number of neutrons in an atom by two.
c. Gamma emission results in no change in atomic number.
d. The atomic number increases with beta minus emission.
e. A nucleon is another term for a metastable radioactive nucleus.

1.14 Concerning radioactivity:

a. A radionuclide decays by a factor of about 1000 in 10 half-lives.
b. A radionuclide with a long half-life poses a lower hazard and fewer constraints are necessary for safe storage than one with a short half-life.
c. A radionuclide may emit both beta and gamma radiation.
d. A becquerel (Bq) is a measure of radioactivity where there is one decay per minute.
e. Specific activity is the radioactivity of unit mass of a radionuclide.

1.15 **The following are true of radioactive material:**

a. A radioactive nucleus must contain an excess of neutrons relative to protons.
b. The half-life is the time for half of the radioactive nuclei in a sample to decay.
c. The half-life is directly proportional to the decay constant.
d. It cannot be inactivated by extreme cooling.
e. The mean lifetime of a nuclide is longer than the half-life.

1.16 **The following statements regarding radionuclides are true:**

a. The effective dose from a radiopharmaceutical is only dependent on the volume to be given to the patient.
b. Each radionuclide emits only one photon energy.
c. Isotopes which emit both beta and gamma radiation are not used for medical purposes, either therapeutically or diagnostically.
d. A gamma-emitting nuclide emits a continuous spectrum of photon energies.
e. The decay constant of an isotope changes according to chemical bonding that may take place with another atom or molecule.

1.17 **Regarding radioactive decay:**

a. The activity of a radionuclide is its rate of decay.
b. The range of a beta particle in water is about 2 cm.
c. Decay occurs at random.
d. Only beta emission is detected by Geiger–Müller counters.
e. The decay constant is the probability of the decay of an atomic nucleus per unit time.

1.1 Answers

a. **True** – these are called rays.
b. **False** – there is less reduction in intensity with distance from a larger source object (e.g. from a patient receiving a dose of a radiopharmaceutical) than from a small source (e.g. from an x-ray tube using a small focal spot).
c. **True** – provided it comes from a point source (and the observer is a few wavelengths distant from the source).
d. **False** – although photons have the properties of both particles and waves, they are not a mixture of the two. In any given measurement they will behave as one or the other.
e. **True** – it may be regarded as a pair of mutually regenerating sinusoidal and oscillating electric and magnetic fields.

1.2 Answers

a. **True** – the constant of proportionality is known as Planck's constant (h) (6.626×10^{-34} Js) where photon energy = h × frequency.
b. **False** – electron volts (eV). Although the joule is a scientifically valid unit (indeed it is the SI standard unit of energy), it gives us an inconveniently small number to deal with for calculations (1 eV = 1.6×10^{-19} joules).
c. **False** – frequency increases with energy. Speed of light in a vacuum is a constant (c = 3×10^8 m s^{-1}).
d. **False** – it moves more slowly when not travelling in a vacuum.
e. **False** – it is not possible to distinguish them in these terms. They are defined by their origin, x-rays from energy changes in orbital electrons and gamma rays from energy changes within the nucleus.

1.3 Answers

a. **True** – wavelength from 400 nm to 700 nm.
b. **True** – wavelength from about 10 mm to 10 m.
c. **False** – sound is a mechanical wave in a medium.
d. **True** – wavelength shorter than 100 nm. All electromagnetic radiation travels at the speed of light in a vacuum and has both quantum and wave properties. Types include radio waves, infrared, visible and ultraviolet light, microwaves, x-rays and gamma radiation.
e. **False** – this is particulate ionising radiation; beta particles are electrons or positrons emitted from a nucleus.

1.4 Answers

a. **False** – medical imaging commonly utilizes x-rays and gamma rays. While beta emission from a scanning nuclide may be tolerated, there are no imaging methods that use beta or alpha particles to form images.

b. **False** – gamma and x-ray radiation are. Neutrons, alpha and beta radiation are not, having a fairly well defined range.

c. **True** – this explains the requirement for radiation protection.

d. **False** – it is only applicable to types of electromagnetic radiation with a short wavelength from a point source in the absence of attenuation. It therefore excludes particulate radiation (e.g. alpha radiation).

e. **True** – while the initial energy transfer is by ionisation, absorption of energy will ultimately be seen as a small temperature rise (about 1°C per 4000 Gy, in water). Heating is insignificant at sublethal doses in tissues, but is a major factor that must be considered in the design of nuclear reactors.

1.5 Answers

a. **False** – it is the sum of the number of protons and neutrons.

b. **True** – and identifies its position on the periodic table.

c. **False** – metastable states are possible, for example technetium-99m and Tc-99.

d. **False** – they are subject to strong binding forces.

e. **True** – it decays to reach a more stable state.

1.6 Answers

a. **False** – nucleons (i.e. protons or neutrons) are components of the nucleus.

b. **False** – not all nuclides are radioactive.

c. **True** – isotopes are nuclides with the same atomic number (protons) but different numbers of neutrons.

d. **False** – see e.

e. **True** – for most nuclides, the combination of neutrons and protons defines their physical properties. Some, such as Tc-99m, require an additional description of their metastable state.

1.7 Answers

a. False – low atomic number nuclei require similar numbers of protons and neutrons to stabilise the nucleus, but at higher atomic numbers more neutrons are required to stabilise a given number of protons (e.g. iodine-127, with 53 protons and 74 neutrons, and lead-208 with 82 protons and 118 neutrons).

b. True – in an element such as tungsten there are more electrons in the L shell than in the K shell and electrons are more likely to be removed from this shell as a result. Therefore a larger number of L x-rays are produced. However, these are of low energy (the L shell binding energy is 12 keV) and are so easily absorbed that they are not seen in the spectrum from a diagnostic x-ray set.

c. False – it is defined as the energy required to completely remove an electron from the influence of an atom. By convention it has a negative value.

d. False – in any atom, the maximum number of electrons in the K shell is two. The number of electrons is equal to the number of protons, so in a helium atom, the K shell accommodates both electrons. The other shells are left empty.

e. True – about 1/1840 relative atomic mass units. Positrons carry positive charge while electrons carry negative charge.

1.8 Answers

a. False – in an atom, electrons can only exist at specific energy levels. Although electrons can jump from one energy level to another (by emitting or absorbing radiation), they cannot exist at energy levels between the shells. The value of these energy levels (K, L, M. etc.) varies according to the nuclide.

b. True – because it is positioned closest to the nucleus and places the orbiting electrons in this shell under the greatest influence of the positive charge of the nucleus.

c. False – it is the outermost shell and is involved in chemical reactions.

d. False – K shell binding energy increases with atomic number (e.g. aluminium Z = 13, K shell 1.6 keV, tungsten Z = 74, k shell 69.5 keV).

e. True – for example only eight electrons may occupy the L shell and 18 may occupy the M shell.

1.9   Answers

a. False – cathode rays are electrons and travel from the negative cathode to the positive anode.

b. True – only a small proportion of the energy is used to produce x-rays.

c. True – because they carry an electrical charge. This effect is used in the focusing cup, and in the electronic focusing in image intensifiers.

d. False – energy units are, by definition, interchangeable since they all measure the same quantity. The electron volt (with its multiples) is a convenient magnitude for measuring energies for all particles and photons, though rather small for everyday purposes. It would take about 10^{24} eV to boil a kettle.

e. False – any atoms or molecules of gas present in the tube could scatter electrons and change the pattern of current flow across the tube.

1.10   Answers

a. True – e.g. technetium-99m conversion to Tc-99 with accompanying gamma emission.

b. False – a proton combines with an orbital K shell electron to produce a neutron. Atomic number decreases by 1.

c. True – gamma radiation released from the nucleus is absorbed by K shell electrons. This photoelectric interaction results in the production of characteristic x-rays. There is no change in the number of nucleons within the nucleus.

d. False – a proton in the nucleus becomes a neutron by releasing a positron. Atomic number decreases by 1.

e. True – this is an artefact demonstrated in magnetic resonance imaging.

1.11   Answers

a. True.

b. True.

c. True.

d. False – decay is not accompanied by this kind of radiation. Bremsstrahlung is caused by interactions of electrons with the electric fields around nuclei and is not a direct consequence of the decay process.

e. True – with either K shell capture or internal conversion.

1.12 Answers

    a. False – the atomic number defines the element and must be the same for all nuclides of the same element.

    b. True – this varies according to the number of additional neutrons present, which may be greater or less than the number required for stability.

    c. True – since this is determined by the atomic number.

    d. False – they may be stable, e.g. carbon-12.

    e. False – e.g. iodine-123 emits gamma rays at 160 keV while iodine-131 emits gamma rays at 360 keV (frequency and energy are proportional).

1.13 Answers

    a. True – they decay by isomeric transition and this may be an appreciable time after the initial decay from the parent to the metastable daughter nuclide.

    b. True – the emission of a helium nucleus removes two neutrons and two protons from the parent nuclide.

    c. True – a change in atomic number requires the emission of a charged particle.

    d. True – a neutron changes into a proton and an electron. The net number of nucleons remains constant.

    e. False – it is the collective term for protons and neutrons.

1.14 Answers

    a. True – it will decay by a factor of 2^{10}, or 1024 (the factor is 2^n, where n is the number of half-lives).

    b. False – the longer time taken to decay to a negligible activity means that long half-life materials generally pose more problems. If equal activities (Bq) rather than equal numbers of atoms (mole) are compared then the longer half-life nuclide will always be more hazardous.

    c. True – gamma emission often accompanies beta decay.

    d. False – a becquerel is one disintegration per second.

    e. True – it can be measured in MBq/mg (or Bq/g).

1.15 Answers

a. False – although beta decay tends to occur if there is an excess of neutrons, there are other forms of decay. In electron capture or positron emission a nucleus with an excess of protons will covert a proton into a neutron to achieve stability.

b. True – the half-life of a radioactive nuclide is the time taken for its radioactivity to reduce to half its original value. Decay is an exponential process.

c. False – they are inversely proportional. Half-life = $\log_e 2$/decay constant.

d. True – radioactive decay is not dependent on physical conditions.

e. True – the mean lifetime is the time taken to decay to $1/e$ (1/2.7182) of the initial activity. The mean lifetime is 1/(decay constant), so it is (half-life)/($\log_e 2$), or about 1.44 times the half-life.

1.16 Answers

a. False – the effective dose from a radiopharmaceutical depends on activity, type of emissions and rate of elimination from the body.

b. False – e.g. cobalt-60 emits 1.117 and 1.332 MeV photons and iodine-131 emits 0.364 and 0.6 MeV photons. In fact, most radionuclides emit gamma rays at several energies.

c. False – iodine-131 can be used for imaging and treatment of thyroid carcinoma.

d. False – the radiation emitted is at specific energies corresponding to energy levels present in the nucleus. X-rays produced during decay are all characteristic and also have specific energy levels.

e. False – it remains constant. Decay is caused by processes in the nucleus, whereas chemical bonding occurs between the outer electron shells.

1.17 Answers

a. True – the units are becquerels (Bq) measuring disintegrations per second.

b. False – 0.2 cm for high energy beta radiation.

c. True – the disintegration of an atom cannot be predicted. The half-life, or decay constant, tells you the probability of decay.

d. False – they can also detect gamma rays, x-rays and alpha particles, depending on the design of the detector.

e. True – the decay constant is the fraction of nuclei decaying per unit time. This is the same as the probability of one atom decaying in unit time. However it is not possible to predict exactly when an individual atom will decay.

2. Production of x-rays

2.1 **When considering characteristic x-ray peaks:**

a. Those for tungsten occur at 17.4 and 19.6 keV.
b. K alpha and K beta peaks refer to transitions from L to K and M to K shells respectively.
c. Their initial cause is a photon–electron interaction within the anode target.
d. They are produced in order to allow an atom to return to a stable energy state.
e. They will not be present in the photon beam from a tungsten target where the tube potential is set at 50 kV.

2.2 **In a general radiography x-ray tube:**

a. The choice of the atomic number of the target affects the characteristic radiation produced.
b. The quantity of bremsstrahlung produced increases with the atomic number of the target.
c. The intensity of x-rays produced is directly proportional to the kV.
d. The intensity of x-rays produced is directly proportional to the mA.
e. Characteristic x-ray peaks make a major contribution to the x-ray beam produced by a tungsten target at high kV.

2.3 **Regarding the spectrum of an x-ray beam:**

a. It has a maximum energy determined by the kVp setting for the tube.
b. It has a maximum energy which is independent of the atomic number of the target.
c. Characteristic peaks are only produced if the tube provides electrons with energy exceeding the K edge energy of the anode material.
d. It is not modified by the amount of filtration employed, as this only influences beam intensity.
e. At a constant kilovoltage, tube current does not affect the maximum or minimum photon energy.

2.4 A diagnostic x-ray tube:

a. May have an anode backed with either molybdenum or carbon to decrease the total heat capacity of the anode.
b. May be so efficient that most of the electrical energy is converted into x-rays.
c. May be fitted with an ionisation chamber.
d. Uses electric fields to control the focal spot size.
e. Has an anode stem that is a poor heat conductor.

2.5 Regarding the x-ray tube:

a. Stationary anodes are no longer used because of safety concerns regarding tube loading.
b. Tube and filament current are of the same magnitude.
c. A stationary anode is necessary for high output requirements.
d. Impairment of the vacuum does not affect the tube current.
e. Because the beam is directed from the anode out of the tube window, shielding is only required on the exit window side of the tube.

2.6 In an x-ray tube:

a. Used in medical diagnostic practice the efficiency of x-ray production is about 10%.
b. The intensity of the radiation depends on anode/cathode distance.
c. The intensity of the radiation depends on the atomic number of the target material.
d. The quality of x-rays generated depends primarily on the kVp and voltage waveform.
e. Increasing the kV increases the wavelength of the radiation.

2.7 The anode heel effect:

a. Is caused by attenuation of x-ray photons at the anode's surface.
b. Is inconvenient and of no practical use.
c. Is more noticeable at larger focus film distances.
d. Is more noticeable with a smaller film.
e. Is more pronounced in a direction parallel to the anode–cathode axis than at right angles to it.

2.8 In rotating anode tubes:

a. The anode diameter is typically 100 mm.
b. Increasing anode diameter increases the tube rating.
c. The target surface is angled to direct the x-ray beam.
d. Heat loss depends on thermal conduction to the tube envelope.
e. The rotor bearings are lubricated with silver.

2.9 Tungsten is used for the target of most x-ray tubes in preference to other materials because:

a. The anode heel effect is not as noticeable compared with other materials.
b. The bremsstrahlung process is more efficient.
c. It has a high thermal conductivity.
d. It has a very high melting point.
e. It is inexpensive.

2.10 In a diagnostic x-ray tube target:

a. Tungsten produces shorter wavelength x-rays than molybdenum given the same kV and current.
b. A stationary anode consists of a tungsten plate backed onto copper.
c. Rhenium decreases surface pitting on a tungsten anode.
d. The heel effect can be completely eliminated in modern tubes.
e. Tungsten anode temperatures exceeding 2500°C are typical during an exposure.

2.11 The following statements are true of the cathode in an x-ray tube:

a. Electrons are formed by thermal transmission.
b. Two filaments may be placed within the same focusing cup.
c. The filament has a low resistance.
d. The focusing cup has a negative potential.
e. The filament has a negative potential.

2.12 Regarding an x-ray tube filament, which of the following are correct:

a. Space charge is formed by tungsten atoms evaporating from the wire.
b. Tungsten is often alloyed with other metals.
c. A minimum filament temperature must be exceeded before a tube current will flow.
d. Tungsten is used because it has a high atomic number.
e. Molybdenum is used as the filament in mammography x-ray tubes.

2.13 The filament is a coil of tungsten because:

a. It is ductile.
b. It has a low melting point.
c. It produces a large amount of bremsstrahlung at the standard filament voltages used.
d. It releases a large thermionic emission.
e. It has a high vapour pressure.

2.14 **Compared to a single phase generator, a high frequency generator allows:**

a. Shorter exposure times.
b. Less variation in kV during an exposure.
c. A larger radiation dose to the patient for a comparable film exposure.
d. The operation of a high speed anode.
e. A lower quality beam to be produced.

2.15 **Regarding x-ray generators:**

a. Capacitor discharge x-ray generators discharge at constant kV.
b. High tension transformers provide the accelerating voltage across the tube.
c. High tension transformers are immersed in oil for insulation and cooling.
d. The variable kV across an x-ray tube is achieved by an autotransformer.
e. X-rays can only be produced using a direct, rather than alternating, potential across a tube.

2.16 **X-ray beam intensity:**

a. Is directly proportional to the tube current.
b. Is not related to the filament current.
c. Is always proportional to the kVp squared.
d. Depends on the voltage waveform.
e. A greater maximum beam intensity is possible from a rotating anode than from a stationary anode.

2.17 **The intensity of the radiation from an x-ray tube is dependent on:**

a. Focal spot size when kV and mA are constant.
b. Choice of anode material.
c. Beam filtration.
d. The distance from the focal spot.
e. Collimation of the beam.

2.18 **Increasing the kV across an x-ray tube with adjustment of mAs to produce the same degree of film blackening:**

a. Increases the x-ray output.
b. Decreases the proportion of scattered to primary radiation at the image receptor.
c. Increases the skin dose to the patient.
d. Decreases the exposure latitude.
e. Increases the mAs required.

2.19   **Increasing tube kV, with all other factors constant:**

a. Increases dose to the patient.
b. Produces a lighter film.
c. Increases radiographic contrast.
d. Shifts the peak of the curve for the x-ray spectrum towards the high energy end of the spectrum.
e. More scatter reaches the film.

2.20   **When tube potential increases:**

a. There is an increase in the relative proportion of photoelectric interactions.
b. There is an increase in the total number of Compton interactions.
c. The patient exit dose increases approximately to the fourth power of the kVp.
d. The dose area product remains roughly constant.
e. The patient dose increases.

2.21   **The half value layer of an x-ray beam will be increased by:**

a. Increasing tube current.
b. Reducing the anode–cathode distance.
c. Increasing the focus–object distance.
d. Increasing exposure time.
e. Increasing the depth of the target layer on the anode.

2.22   **Concerning x-ray beam quality:**

a. It is affected by the applied voltage waveform.
b. It is unrelated to tube kV.
c. HVL increases with greater tube filtration.
d. It is not defined simply by half value thickness.
e. As a result of beam hardening the HVL approaches a constant value with each additional HVL of filtration.

2.23   **Filtration of x-rays:**

a. Hardens the beam.
b. Increases the number of photons in the beam.
c. Reduces the entrance surface dose.
d. Aluminium is useful because its K edge does not interfere with the spectrum.
e. The inherent filtration component is typically 0.5–1 mm aluminium for a diagnostic x-ray tube.

2.24 **The following are true of filtration:**

a. Inherent filtration includes the borosilicate tube window, cooling oil and the tube casing but not the light beam diaphragm mirror.
b. Aluminium must be used.
c. For general diagnostic use the total filtration of an x-ray set should be 1.5 mm of aluminium.
d. A rhodium backing is added to the molybdenum disc to absorb its characteristic radiation in mammography.
e. Compound filters are no longer used in radiology.

2.25 **An x-ray tube rating chart depicts the maximum permissible combination of kVp, mA (average current) and time during an x-ray exposure. The following factors may influence the shape of a tube rating chart:**

a. Design of filament.
b. Size of the patient.
c. Speed of anode rotation.
d. Efficiency of cooling mechanisms.
e. The x-ray generator type.

2.26 **The following statements are true regarding the maximum rating of an x-ray tube:**

a. For short exposure times it is limited by heating of the anode surface by bombardment with high energy electrons.
b. For short exposure times it depends upon the average value of the voltage waveform across the tube.
c. For long exposure times it is limited by the total amount of heat which accumulates in the anode.
d. In a modern angiography system active anode cooling mechanisms allow the use of longer exposure runs.
e. The maximum rating of a modern CT x-ray tube is 500 000 heat units.

2.1 Answers

a. **False** – these are the peaks for molybdenum.
b. **True**.
c. **False** – the initial interaction is a collision between an electron produced by the filament and a bound electron in the target, ejecting the bound electron from its shell.
d. **True** – the removal of an inner shell electron promotes the atom to a higher energy state. This energy is removed by the emission of an x-ray photon when the vacancy in the inner shell electron shell is filled with an outer shell electron.
e. **True** – they are only present when the tube potential provides electrons with energy that exceeds that of the K shell binding energy (i.e. 69.5 keV for tungsten).

2.2 Answers

a. **True** – the energy of the characteristic radiation depends on the energy difference in electron shells and is determined by the atomic number (Z). The shape of the bremsstrahlung spectrum is unaffected by Z.
b. **True** – the stronger electric field associated with higher atomic number nuclei means that x-ray-producing interactions are more likely.
c. **False** – output is approximately proportional to the square of the kV.
d. **True** – more electrons strike the target, so more x-ray photons are produced.
e. **False** – only about 10% of the beam intensity is derived from characteristic radiation between 80 and 150 kV.

2.3 Answers

a. **True** – minimum wavelength (or maximum energy) of beam is determined by the maximum energy of the electrons striking the target, which depends on the kV across the tube.
b. **True** – target material does not affect the maximum photon energy.
c. **True** – L shell x-rays are produced if the electron energy exceeds the L edge, but these have a very low energy and do not contribute to the spectrum emerging from the tube.
d. **False** – filtration tends to remove low energy photons thereby reducing intensity, hardening the beam and increasing the mean beam energy of the spectrum.
e. **True** – only the number of photons (or intensity) is affected by this.

2.4 Answers

a. **False** – it increases the heat capacity and reduces the mass of the anode. This second factor allows more efficient anode rotation.

b. **False** – x-ray production by bremsstrahlung and photoelectric effect is extremely inefficient at diagnostic energies. Around 99–99.5% of the energy produced is converted into heat with the remaining 0.5–1% converted into x-rays. The process becomes more efficient at higher kilovoltages, outside the diagnostic range.

c. **True** – in the form of a Dose Area Product meter, which measures the product of dose and field size. Appropriate calibration allows it to give a reading, usually in cGy cm^2.

d. **True** – from the focusing cup.

e. **True** – to protect the rotor assembly from heat damage.

2.5 Answers

a. **False** – many portable sets and most dental tubes use stationary anodes.

b. **False** – the filament current is usually 10 to 100 times greater than the tube current (up to 10 A vs. 0.5–1000 mA).

c. **False** – the focal track on the anode of a rotating target is larger than the spot on a stationary target, dissipating the heat over a larger surface, thereby allowing a greater heat loading and therefore a higher output.

d. **False** – the vacuum allows unimpeded electron acceleration. Any impairment of the vacuum will affect tube current and electrical stability.

e. **False** – although the target angle directs the beam through the window, x-rays are produced in all directions from the focal spot. x-rays are also produced from extra focal radiation caused by stray electrons striking the target outside the focal spot. Lead shielding is therefore employed to encase the whole tube excluding the window itself.

2.6 Answers

a. **False** – only 0.5–1%. Efficiency increases with kV and with Z of the target.

b. **False** – this is not relevant.

c. **True** – the resultant x-ray intensity for tungsten is around 10 times greater than aluminium at 100 kV for a set tube current.

d. **True** – the kVp determines the maximum photon energy. The general shape of the bremsstrahlung spectrum is affected by the voltage waveform and the beam filtration.

e. **False** – as kV increases both the peak and mean photon energy increase. Therefore wavelength decreases according to $E = hc/\lambda$ (where λ is wavelength, h is Planck's constant and c is speed of light).

2.7 Answers

a. **True** – photons exiting the target at an oblique angle must traverse a greater thickness of material than those exiting at right angles to the surface. The anode heel effect can be ignored in much conventional x-ray work, though it is important in the design of mammographic x-ray tubes. It can affect the practical measurement of kV, which uses the difference in signal from two differently filtered radiation detectors. Care is needed to avoid spurious readings arising from intensity differences caused by the heel effect.

b. **False** – it is utilised in mammography and x-rays of large body parts.

c. **False** – because there is greater divergence of the beam, the film will only intercept the central portion of the field.

d. **False** – a larger film will show the effect more easily. A small film will only intercept the central portion of the field.

e. **True** – because of the angulation of the target, there is a much greater variation in the angle at which photons exit the target parallel to the anode–cathode axis.

2.8 Answers

a. **True**.

b. **True** – a larger target area is offered to the electron beam, which decreases the heat deposition per unit area and increases the rating.

c. **True** – and the degree of angulation determines the focal spot size.

d. **False** – the main method of heat loss is radiation to the tube envelope.

e. **True** – other lubricants, such as oil, would evaporate in the vacuum within the envelope.

2.9 Answers

a. **False** – all anode materials are affected by this problem.

b. **True** – the intensity of the resulting x-ray beam is high because of its high atomic number.

c. **True** – this allows heat to be conducted away from the focal spot.

d. **True** – 3370°C. Also tungsten has a high thermal conductivity, a low vapour pressure and good mechanical properties for anode construction.

e. **False** – it is not, but this is not the primary concern. Physical properties are more important.

2.10 Answers

a. **False** – the applied voltage and its waveform alone determine this.
b. **True** – because copper has a higher thermal storage capacity than tungsten alone and copper is a better heat conductor, which dissipates heat away from the target.
c. **True** – it is alloyed with tungsten for this purpose to prolong the lifetime of the tube.
d. **False** – the physical processes involved cannot be designed out.
e. **True** – to over 3000°C.

2.11 Answers

a. **False** – heating of the filament by a large current allows electrons to boil off and produce a space charge around the cathode. This can then be accelerated towards the anode to produce x-rays. The process is called thermionic emission.
b. **True** – but they are usually separate.
c. **False** – high resistance is required to generate the heat needed to produce thermionic emission of electrons.
d. **True** – focusing uses a negative cup potential to repel electrons from the filament and produces a narrower beam. The focusing cup is part of the cathode block.
e. **True** – but the cup normally has a more negative potential than the filament.

2.12 Answers

a. **False** – electrons are released from the wire to form the space charge.
b. **False**.
c. **True** – the threshold for thermionic emission is 2200°C.
d. **False** – this is why it is used as a target.
e. **False** – tungsten is used.

2.13 Answers

a. **True**.
b. **False**.
c. **False** – the filament does not emit radiation (but the anode does).
d. **True**.
e. **False** – because it is ductile, has good thermionic emission properties relative to other elements, a high melting point and a low vapour pressure.

2.14 Answers

a. True – because there is less ripple the tube potential is closer to the peak kV for a greater proportion of the exposure. This increases both the x-ray output and the mean photon energy.

b. True – this is the reason for the higher tube output.

c. False – more high energy photons are produced as a fraction of the total x-rays in a high frequency generator. There is less ripple in the voltage supplied to the tube and therefore less dose to the patient (as dose is more dependent on low energy photons).

d. False – the kV waveform and anode speed are independent of each other.

e. False – the kV ripple from a single phase full rectified beam is 100% versus 13% for a three-phase generator and approaching zero for a high frequency generator. As beam quality is determined by the average kV the last will be superior.

2.15 Answers

a. False – the tube kV falls as the capacitor releases stored charge. The fall in kV depends on the tube current and exposure time (mAs).

b. True – this is for the tube voltage.

c. True – oil is an excellent electrical insulator.

d. True – there are variable tappings on the autotransformer, which selects a voltage to be fed to the high tension transformer from the mains voltage.

e. False – some simple x-ray sets are self rectifying. The reverse phase of the supply is also applied to the tube, but no current flows during this phase because there is no thermionic emission from the anode. An alternating potential will reduce the average current across the tube.

2.16 Answers

a. True – intensity is defined as the energy per unit area per unit time – or the number of photons times the mean energy per unit area per unit time. If all other conditions stay the same, the rate of x-ray production will depend on the rate at which electrons strike the target. The tube current (mA) is a direct measure of this.

b. False – tube current increases with filament current. However the relationship is not linear, and the tube current tends to rise in greater increments with small increases in the filament current.

c. False – increasing the kV increases both the range of photon energies and the number of photons produced at each energy, and this gives rise to an approximate kV squared relationship. The exact relationship will depend on waveform and filtration. At the low tube potentials used in mammography, the relationship is closer to kV cubed.

d. **True** – a waveform with a small ripple will be at a value close to the peak voltage for most of the time. The electrons will have a higher mean energy and this will result in both more x-ray photons and a greater mean photon energy.

e. **True** – because of the higher heat rating, which allows larger maximum tube currents to be used.

2.17 Answers

a. **False** – this has no relation to intensity.

b. **True** – higher atomic number targets produce more bremsstrahlung for a given kV and mAs. This is because larger nuclei have stronger electric fields, which are more effective at deflecting the incoming electrons. The electron's deflection causes it to lose energy in the form of x-rays.

c. **True** – increased filtration reduces beam intensity, while at the same time hardening the beam. Changing the filter material will also affect the absorption of photons from the spectrum and change intensity.

d. **True** – intensity will fall with increasing distance from the focal spot, according to the inverse square law.

e. **False** – while this reduces the total number of photons (and the dose area product), the intensity of the remaining part of the beam remains the same.

2.18 Answers

a. **False** – the exposure (mAs) will be reduced to compensate for the increased kV.

b. **False** – at higher tube voltage, x-rays are more penetrating and scattering events will, on average, occur at a greater depth in the patient and closer to the film. The scattered photons will also, on average, be more penetrating. These two effects will tend to increase the proportion of scattered radiation in the image.

c. **False** – for the same film blackening the skin dose is reduced. For example, going from 70 to 80 kV requires approximate halving of the mAs to produce the same film blackening. This would lead to an increase of $(80/70)^2$ (about 30%) in output per mAs, but a 50% reduction in mAs, which gives an overall reduction in dose of 35%.

d. **False** – exposure latitude is defined as the range of exposure factors that will give a correctly exposed image of the subject. This will be increased as kV increases. The higher mean photon energy reduces subject contrast, which means that the range of film exposure is reduced. A smaller part of the straight portion of the characteristic curve of the film is used as a result. The exposure can therefore be in error to a greater extent, without producing densities outside the useful range.

e. **False** – the increased output per mAs and the more penetrating radiation, due to the increased tube kV, requires the exposure (mAs) to be reduced (see c).

2.19 Answers

a. **True** – beam intensity will increase proportional to kV squared.
b. **False** – greater exposure results in greater film density.
c. **False** – contrast decreases with higher kV.
d. **True** – it increases the mean energy of the x-ray photons.
e. **True** – the increased x-ray output increases the total amount of scatter. The scattered photons are also on average more penetrating. Both of these factors allow more scattered photons to reach the film.

2.20 Answers

a. **False** – photoelectric interactions are favoured at lower photon energies.
b. **True** – Compton interactions are favoured at a higher kV, and increasing the kV increases the total number of photons.
c. **True** – the x-ray output increases with kV squared. As the x-ray beam passes through the patient the mean energy of the beam increases due to filtration. As a result the kVp dependence increases to a fourth power law.
d. **False** – dose area product is related to beam intensity. As beam intensity is related to kVp squared, dose area product will increase.
e. **True** – unless the mAs is reduced to produce the same photographic density.

2.21 Answers

a. **False** – there is no effect on quality, only on intensity.
b. **False** – this has no effect.
c. **False** – assuming that x-ray absorption in air is negligible.
d. **False** – this has no effect.
e. **False** – this has no effect.

2.22 Answers

a. **True** – a generator with small kV ripple will operate close to the peak kV for a greater proportion of the time than one with a large kV ripple. The mean photon energy will be higher and the beam will be more penetrating.
b. **False** – both the peak and mean photon energy are dependent on tube potential (kV).
c. **True** – added filtration hardens the beam.
d. **True** – although beam quality is a description of the penetrating power of the radiation, it is only partially described by the first HVL. The same HVL could result from different combinations of generating potential and filtration, so a full description requires detailed information on the radiation spectrum.
e. **True** – the HVL will tend towards a constant value as the thickness of absorber increases.

2.23 Answers

a. True – hardening is defined as an increase in the penetrating power of the beam, as measured by the HVL. Filtration hardens the beam by preferentially removing lower energy photons.

b. False – because some photons are removed, the total number in the beam will be reduced.

c. True – by removing low energy photons that contribute to dose but not image formation.

d. True – this prevents x-rays being absorbed by the filter at a photon energy that is needed for image formation. The K edge of aluminium is 1.6 keV.

e. True – inherent filtration is that which derives from the tube components, rather than from material deliberately added to modify the spectrum.

2.24 Answers

a. False – as the light beam diaphragm mirror also attenuates the x-ray beam.

b. False – mammography uses rhodium and molybdenum filters, while CT scanning may use copper filtration.

c. False – 1.5 mm should be the minimum, non-removable component of the filtration. X-ray equipment usually has filtration appropriate to the maximum kV at which it can operate, and this means at least 2.5 mm for most diagnostic sets. It is quite unusual for the operator to vary the filtration with kV, so most tubes have a fixed amount (about 3 mm) of filtration.

d. False – compound filters are not used in mammography.

e. False – copper and aluminium filters are used in CT scanners.

2.25 Answers

a. True.

b. False – although this may require an increase in the exposure factors it will not determine the maximum combination of mA, kVp and time.

c. True – and size of the anode.

d. True.

e. True.

2.26 Answers

a. **True**.

b. **False** – it is limited by peak instantaneous power delivery at the anode surface and the maximum anode surface temperature which results. This is largely set by the peak value of the voltage waveform.

c. **True** – this can be calculated from the average power delivered over the exposure time, plus the influence of anode cooling processes. Therefore it is the average (or effective) kilovoltage, and not peak kV, which becomes significant.

d. **True** – cooling the tube using active circulation of oil in the tube housing and air conditioning improves heat dissipation from the anode by cooling the x-ray tube housing. The anode also tends to have a larger mass to allow greater heat storage.

e. **False** – because of the enormous amount of heat generated by the long exposures used in spiral scanning for volume acquisition, the anodes must have a rating of several million heat units.

3. Interactions of ionising radiation with matter

3.1 **Regarding attenuation of a diagnostic x-ray beam:**

a. Total attenuation is the sum of attenuations from Compton, elastic and photoelectric effects.

b. It is the fractional reduction in intensity of a primary beam through a medium.

c. It is related to the atomic number of the absorbing material.

d. By the addition of a series of aluminium filters of equal thickness, the beam intensity would be attenuated by equal fractions.

e. Attenuation is related to the inverse square law.

3.2 **Concerning attenuation when a diagnostic x-ray beam interacts with matter:**

a. It is the absorption of radiation in matter.

b. Scatter is a cause of attenuation.

c. It increases with the thickness of the attenuating object.

d. Increasing photon energy always leads to a steady reduction in beam attenuation.

e. It is related to the temperature of a fixed mass of attenuating material.

3.3 **X-rays from diagnostic x-ray generators may participate in the following processes:**

a. Compton scatter.

b. Linear acceleration.

c. Pair production.

d. Elastic scatter.

e. Bremsstrahlung production.

3.4 **Attenuation of a monoenergetic photon beam can lead to:**

a. Deflection of photons through more than 90° with an increase in their energy.

b. Beam hardening.

c. Deflection of photons, which retain all their energy.

d. Electromagnetic induction.

e. The production of characteristic radiation.

3.5 **The mass attenuation coefficient:**

a. Is derived from the linear attenuation coefficient (LAC) multiplied by the density.
b. Is interchangeable with the LAC.
c. Is a more important quantity than LAC in radiology.
d. For water as liquid, vapour and ice is identical.
e. Is measured per unit volume.

3.6 **The linear attenuation coefficient of water:**

a. Has a value of 35 mm at 60 keV.
b. Depends on the mAs setting.
c. Is higher than that of fat.
d. Generally decreases as photon energy increases.
e. Is the fractional reduction in intensity per unit thickness.

3.7 **Practical applications of the linear attenuation coefficient include:**

a. To calculate the thickness of shielding required for the walls of a fluoroscopy suite.
b. Assigning Hounsfield units to a pixel in a CT image.
c. Grey scale allocation of structures in a chest x-ray.
d. Calculating the total scatter produced from a single exposure.
e. Determining the half value layer of an x-ray beam.

3.8 **The half value thickness of water for a 60 keV monoenergetic photon beam is 35 mm. Therefore:**

a. A 30 keV beam would have a half value layer of less than 35 mm.
b. In 35 cm of water the beam would be reduced to around 1%.
c. 70 mm of water would attenuate the beam by 90%.
d. The half value thickness of bone will be a lower value.
e. For an x-ray unit working at 60 kVp, the half value layer would be more than 35 mm.

3.9 **Concerning the photoelectric effect:**

a. It involves an unbound electron.
b. It occurs with a probability which increases in direct proportion with the energy of the photon.
c. The incident photon energy is all converted into kinetic energy of the electron.
d. The photoelectric contribution to the mass attenuation coefficient increases roughly as the cube of atomic number.
e. It causes ionisation of the atom.

3.10 Concerning the photoelectric effect of x-ray photons:

a. The K absorption edge threshold occurs at an energy that exceeds that of K shell characteristic x-rays.
b. Photoelectric absorption results in characteristic x-ray production.
c. It may occur with electron shells other than the K shell.
d. The probability of such an interaction increases with increasing photon energy.
e. It may result in scattered radiation.

3.11 The photoelectric effect:

a. Results in total absorption of incident photon energy.
b. Only occurs above a set electromagnetic wave frequency.
c. Increases with kV.
d. Is a separate phenomenon to K edge absorption in intensifying screens.
e. Accounts for most of the patient dose in diagnostic x-ray imaging.

3.12 Practical applications relying on the photoelectric effect alone include:

a. The anode heel effect.
b. Photographic exposure.
c. Dose area product meters.
d. Rare earth filters.
e. Thermoluminescent dose meters.

3.13 Regarding scatter:

a. More is produced by the photoelectric effect than the Compton effect.
b. The contribution of x-ray scatter incident upon an image receptor reduces spatial resolution.
c. Scatter increases the signal to noise ratio.
d. Scatter reaching the image receptor increases when a higher kV is used.
e. Scattered x-rays escaping a patient during a barium enema examination result in a negligible radiation hazard to staff.

3.14 **In Compton scattering:**

   a. The whole of the photon energy may be transferred to the recoil electron.
   b. The amount of scattering of x-rays that occurs depends on the electron density of the scattering material.
   c. The recoil electrons of maximum energy are those in the same direction as the incident photon.
   d. More scatter is measured on the tube side of the patient at normal diagnostic energies than on the film side.
   e. Increasing the object–film distance reduces the amount of scatter reaching the film.

3.15 **In the Compton effect:**

   a. A photon interacts with a free electron.
   b. Incident photon energy is shared between an electron and the nucleus.
   c. The effective atomic number of the object determines the amount of scatter produced.
   d. Scatter is proportional to electron density.
   e. An incident photon of high energy will lose more energy than a low energy photon in a Compton interaction with an electron at a given angle.

3.16 **Concerning the Compton effect:**

   a. The reduction in energy of the scattered photon is greater with larger angles of scatter.
   b. An incident photon can have the same energy as a scattered photon.
   c. It produces photoelectrons.
   d. Part of the incident photon energy is transferred to an outer shell electron and part becomes scattered radiation.
   e. It does not occur in bone at low kV.

3.17 **Regarding scattered radiation in diagnostic radiology:**

   a. The change in wavelength of an x-ray photon depends mainly on the structure of the tissue causing the scatter.
   b. Most scattered photons emerging from a patient are in the forward direction.
   c. At increased kV more photons are deflected through large angles.
   d. It is decreased in amount by collimation of the x-ray beam.
   e. Increasing the focus–film distance (with the same object–film distance) will increase total quantity of scatter events at a set tube mAs and kV.

3.1 Answers

a. **False** – the attenuation coefficient is the sum of the coefficients from the different processes, but the total attenuation is the product of the attenuation from each process.
b. **True** – this is the definition of attenuation.
c. **True** – as the probability of photoelectric absorption is proportional to Z cubed.
d. **False** – this would be true only if the attenuation were truly exponential, as occurs with a monoenergetic beam.
e. **False** – the inverse square law describes reduction in intensity caused by divergence of the beam from a point. Attenuation describes the reduction in intensity caused by interactions with matter.

3.2 Answers

a. **False** – it is a combination of absorption and scatter.
b. **True** – via the Compton interaction.
c. **True** – the longer the path of the beam, the greater the probability of an interaction taking place.
d. **False** – generally this is true, except for the special case of increasing photon energy just beyond a K shell absorption edge. In this instance the degree of attenuation increases discontinuously when photon energy exceeds the K shell energy threshold.
e. **False** – this is unrelated so long as the mass of material is fixed. If only the volume of material is fixed, e.g. air in an unsealed ionisation chamber, temperature will affect the attenuation.

3.3 Answers

a. **True**.
b. **False** – this is the process where electrons are accelerated to very high energies to produce high energy therapeutic x-rays (radiotherapy).
c. **False** – when a high energy photon (>1.02 MeV) approaches a nucleus it may be converted into a positron and an electron. This photon energy cannot be achieved at the tube voltages used in diagnostic radiology.
d. **True** – elastic scatter is an interaction causing deflection of the incoming photon with no resultant loss of energy.
e. **False** – this is an electron interaction.

3.4 Answers

a. False – photons cannot gain energy through the Compton process.

b. False – in fact as a result of scatter the exit beam will have a wider energy range and will be 'softer'. A beam with a spectrum of energies would be hardened by filtration.

c. True – elastic scattering, accounting for about 5% of total scatter in diagnostic radiology.

d. False – this is when a magnetic field is induced around a wire with a current flowing through it, or when a current is induced in a wire by a varying magnetic field.

e. True – by photoelectric interactions.

3.5 Answers

a. False – LAC divided by density.

b. False – mass attenuation coefficient describes the attenuation by a unit mass of material per unit area. The LAC describes attenuation by a unit thickness of material.

c. False – the film density resulting from the attenuation of a certain thickness of an object is more meaningful than the mass of tissue producing the effect.

d. True – since the individual water molecules are identical, what matters is how many of them attenuate the beam. By dividing the LAC by the density, only the quantity of material in the beam is considered. If the material is the same (e.g. ice, water and steam) the mass attenuation coefficient is the same.

e. False – meters squared per kilogram.

3.6 Answers

a. False – this is the half value layer. Linear attenuation coefficient would be expressed in mm^{-1}. Incorrect units are a good guide to a false question.

b. False – the LAC is a property of the material and the radiation energy. It is completely unrelated to mAs.

c. True – it increases with atomic number and with increasing physical density. Fat produces less attenuation than water.

d. True – except for absorption edges. The probability of photoelectric interactions decreases with increasing photon energy, and this causes the LAC to decrease.

e. True – this is its definition.

3.7 Answers

a. **True** – by knowing the radiation transmission through a protective barrier, the thickness of lead, concrete or barium plaster required for x-ray room shielding can be calculated.

b. **True** – the LAC of a pixel is related to that of water before a Hounsfield unit is allocated to it.

c. **True** – differential attenuation of x-rays in individual tissues leads to separate corresponding densities in the radiograph.

d. **False** – this is the Compton contribution to the LAC.

e. **True** – HVL =$\log_e$ 2/LAC (where the LAC is taken from that of a monoenergetic beam of the same mean energy).

3.8 Answers

a. **True** – because the linear attenuation coefficient will be greater (i.e. there will be greater attenuation per unit distance at lower energy).

b. **False** – beam intensity is reduced to around 1000th of its original value with 10 half value thicknesses.

c. **False** – 75% (70 mm is two half value thicknesses).

d. **True** – because of the greater amount of attenuation per unit length.

e. **False** – the kVp is the maximum potential achieved by the tube, so the electron energy in keV will have a maximum value numerically equal to the kVp . The x-rays produced have a spectrum of energies with a peak at about a half to one third of the electron energy. The average energy of the beam is therefore significantly lower than 60 keV, and the beam would require less water to reduce its intensity by half.

3.9 Answers

a. **False** – it involves a bound inner shell electron.

b. **False** – the probability of photoelectric interactions varies inversely with the cube of the energy.

c. **False** – some energy is lost in overcoming the binding energy of the electron.

d. **True** – photoelectric effect is proportional to Z cubed.

e. **True** – as an electron is removed a net positive charge results.

3.10 Answers

a. **True** – an electron falling from the L or M shell has a defined binding energy. The energy released (in the form of a characteristic x-ray) is the difference between the binding energies of the two shells. This is slightly less than the energy needed to remove an electron from the K shell.

b. **True** – the ejected inner shell photoelectron is replaced by an outer shell electron. The electron must lose energy in the process of becoming more tightly bound to the nucleus, and achieves this by emitting an x-ray photon.

c. **True** – L shell electrons can also produce these interactions because they also have a sufficient binding energy to be considered 'bound'. It can also occur with outer shell electrons but not using x-rays. The photon energy at which this occurs is in the ultraviolet to visible range (i.e. with lower energy).

d. **False** – the probability of photoelectric interactions is inversely proportional to the cube of the photon energy.

e. **False** – scatter is predominantly caused by the Compton effect.

3.11 Answers

a. **True** – hence photoelectric absorption.

b. **True** – the incoming photon must have enough energy, or a high enough frequency, to exceed the binding energy of the electron which it strikes.

c. **False** – the probability of photoelectric interactions decreases with the cube of photon energy. Increased tube potential increases the mean photon energy.

d. **False** – K edge absorption refers to photoelectric interactions that occur with photons at energies above the K shell binding energy in an atom. When the K edge is exceeded there is a sudden increase in the number of photoelectric interactions.

e. **True** – although Compton interactions predominate at some energies and for some tissues, they result in relatively little energy absorption. Photons that undergo Compton scatter are eventually absorbed by photoelectric processes.

3.12 Answers

a. **False**.

b. **True**.

c. **False** – both Compton and photoelectric processes result in ionisation of air, which gives rise to the current measured by the meter.

d. **True** – the spectrum shaping properties of rare earth filters depends on the enhanced absorption of photons by the photoelectric effect, at energies slightly above the K edge.

e. **False** – thermoluminecence depends on raising electrons from the valence band to the conduction band. This is likely to occur through Compton interactions.

3.13 Answers

a. **False** – most scatter is from Compton interactions, while the photoelectric effect is a process of complete absorption.
b. **False** – it decreases subject contrast and signal to noise ratio.
c. **False** – it decreases it.
d. **True** – at higher kV there are a greater proportion of Compton interactions (of the total number of attenuated photons) and more of the scatter is in a forward direction. It is produced closer to the exit surface of the patient and it is more penetrating, which makes it more likely to reach the film.
e. **False** –scatter dose rates near fluoroscopy patients are significant and require radiation protection measures.

3.14 Answers

a. **False** – it is the photon that is scattered. If the photon still exists, it cannot have given all of its energy to the electron. Total absorption occurs in photoelectric interactions.
b. **True** – scatter increases with increasing electron density.
c. **True** – think of the interaction as a snooker shot. Glancing collisions transfer much less energy from the white ball (photon) to the coloured ball (electron).
d. **True** – backscatter is the predominant direction of Compton scatter emerging from the patient at the photon energies used in diagnostic radiology. This is because most of the interactions occur close to the entrance surface of the patient, so that backscattered photons are attenuated less than forward scattered ones. This should not be confused with the direction of scatter from a point target (electron), which becomes increasingly more forward at higher energies.
e. **True** – this is the principle of the air-gap technique, where scattered photons miss the film and are effectively filtered out by the gap to improve image quality.

3.15 Answers

a. **True** – in the outer shell of the atom. The binding energy is so much lower than the photon energy that the electron behaves as though it were free.
b. **False** – the energy donated by the photon goes solely to the electron. The interaction has nothing to do with the nucleus.
c. **False** – the probability of scatter is independent of z.
d. **True** – since the greater the concentration of electrons, the greater the probability of an interaction of a photon and a free electron.
e. **True** – the magnitude of the wavelength shift ($\Delta\lambda$) depends on the scattering angle. (Energy, $E = hc/\lambda$. Energy of scattered photon = $hc/(\lambda + \Delta\lambda)$.) If λ is small, $\Delta\lambda$ has a much greater effect on E, and $\Delta\lambda$ depends only on scattering angle, not on λ.

3.16 Answers

a. **True**.

b. **False** – this is the mechanism in elastic scatter, where the photon energy is absorbed by an electron and then re-emitted at a different angle with the same energy.

c. **False** – these are formed as a result of photoelectric interactions.

d. **True** – this defines a Compton interaction.

e. **False** – it occurs in all tissues, and the proportion of Compton interactions increases with higher kV. However photoelectric interactions predominate under 50 keV.

3.17 Answers

a. **False** – the wavelength shift depends only on the angle of scatter. The photon interacts with a free electron, so the type of material is irrelevant.

b. **False** – more of the forward scattered photons are absorbed within the patient, which explains why more backscatter escapes the patient, but the number of scattering events is about the same in either direction.

c. **False** – there is not much change in the geometric distribution of scatter within the diagnostic range. What change there is tends to increase the proportion of forward (small angle) scatter.

d. **True** – this is one of the main practical measures to reduce scatter.

e. **False** – since the number of photons remains constant (same mAs and kV) the number of scatter events will remain unchanged (if you cone down to keep the field size the same at the increased FFD, then the number of photons is reduced).

4. Factors affecting image quality

4.1 **Extrafocal radiation:**

　　a. In a metal tube can be limited by grounding the metal tube envelope.
　　b. Can be completely removed from the beam by appropriate filtration.
　　c. Is more prominent at low tube currents.
　　d. Has no effect on image quality.
　　e. Is caused by secondary electrons from the target striking the anode outside the target area.

4.2 **The effective focal spot size for a rotating anode:**

　　a. Depends on anode angle.
　　b. Depends on filament size.
　　c. Depends on anode diameter.
　　d. Depends on speed of anode rotation.
　　e. Is smaller than the actual focal spot size.

4.3 **Effective focal spot size:**

　　a. Can be measured by a pinhole camera technique.
　　b. Is decreased by increasing the angle of the anode.
　　c. Is independent of tube current.
　　d. Is independent of tube kV.
　　e. Is dependent on anode rotation speed.

4.4 **Assuming that other factors are optimised, these factors may introduce unsharpness to an image:**

　　a. Short exposures.
　　b. A small focal spot.
　　c. Use of an intensifying screen.
　　d. Use of a double film emulsion.
　　e. A short object–film distance.

4.5 **Radiographic spatial resolution may be improved by:**

　　a. Increasing focus–object distance.
　　b. High subject contrast.
　　c. Using a high output x-ray tube.
　　d. Using an anti-scatter grid.
　　e. Increasing kV.

4.6 **The following factors influence geometric unsharpness:**

a. Focal spot size.
b. Reduced absorption of x-rays near the edge of the subject.
c. Speed of the film–screen combination.
d. Object to film distance.
e. A high kV technique.

4.7 **These statements are true of spatial resolution:**

a. It can be measured directly by imaging a pinhole.
b. It is reduced when an object is geometrically magnified, with a small focal spot.
c. The MTF curve may be used to estimate the limiting resolution of a system.
d. It is significantly better in computed radiology than in film-screen radiography.
e. In fluoroscopy is limited by the electronic band width of the TV camera.

4.8 **Regarding the modulation transfer function (MTF):**

a. The MTF portrays how well signal contrast at different spatial frequencies is reproduced by the imaging system.
b. It contains the same information as the line spread function.
c. Is not affected by quantum mottle.
d. Is the reciprocal of the line spread function.
e. A system cannot resolve the image signal when the MTF is 1.

4.9 **The following are true of the modulation transfer function:**

a. The MTF of a system is the sum of the MTFs of the individual components of the system.
b. The MTF cannot exceed 1.0.
c. Compared to a general radiography system, a mammography system will have a higher MTF value when imaging the same high spatial frequency test object.
d. The MTF of a film–screen combination is dominated by the MTF of the screen.
e. The MTF of a computed radiography system is limited by the diameter of the laser beam that scans the image plate.

4.10 **Modulation transfer function:**

a. Of a film–screen system normally increases with increasing spatial frequency.
b. Is improved by increasing focal spot size.
c. Of a digital image intensifier TV system improves with electronic magnification.
d. Of a film–screen combination depends upon focal spot size.
e. Is around 10% at 1 line pair per millimetre for a gamma camera.

4.11 For an x-ray exposure, scattered radiation reaching a film can be reduced by using these factors alone:

a. Use of a grid.
b. Increasing the field size.
c. Reducing the object–film distance.
d. Increasing the focus-film distance.
e. Breath holding.

4.12 Compton scatter reduces image quality. It can be minimized by:

a. Achieving a higher dose area product reading at the end of the exposure.
b. Compression.
c. Decreasing the kV.
d. Reducing the exposure time while achieving the same degree of film blackening.
e. Lead backing on the cassette.

4.13 Regarding noise in a radiographic image:

a. Structure mottle is more significant than quantum mottle in a fast film–screen combination.
b. Increasing the thickness of the phosphor layer will increase quantum mottle.
c. Quantum mottle is due to the statistical variation in the number of x-ray photons absorbed per unit area.
d. Quantum mottle is made more noticeable with magnification radiography.
e. Noise is made more visible by increasing the contrast control of the display monitor of a fluoroscopy system.

4.14 Quantum mottle is demonstrated by a film–screen combination. This could be caused by:

a. Using a slow film.
b. Uneven light emission from phosphor crystals in the intensifying screen.
c. A fast film–screen combination.
d. Using a tube with a high heat rating.
e. Using an excessively high kV.

4.15 Regarding film viewing conditions:

a. A high level of ambient lighting should be used.
b. Masking uncovered parts of the illuminator makes no difference to the interpretation of the viewed image.
c. The fluorescent tubes in adjacent viewing boxes can be of a slightly different light output and colour temperature.
d. Radiographic contrast is dependent on viewing conditions.
e. Human visual perception responds to light in a linear manner when viewing a radiograph.

4.16 Regarding the latent image on film:

a. The mechanism of production was described by the Gurney and Mott theory.
b. One photon of light energy acting on one film grain provides a developable image.
c. It involves electron transfer through the crystal when electrons gain sufficient energy.
d. Requires the migration of positive silver ions through the interstitial spaces of the crystal.
e. Clumps of silver form at the sensitivity speck.

4.17 Concerning x-ray film:

a. The characteristic curve of a film is a graph of log exposure plotted against the speed of a film.
b. Gamma $= (D_2 - D_1)/\log_{10}(E_2/E_1)$, where exposures E_1 and E_2 produce film densities of D_1 and D_2 on the characteristic curve.
c. A film with high 'gamma' has a high film contrast.
d. The latitude of a film is directly proportional to gamma.
e. The gamma of a film exposed with an intensifying screen is typically 2 to 3.5.

4.18 Regarding contrast:

a. Subjective (perceived) contrast may be defined as the relative light intensity of various parts of the radiographic image as perceived by an observer.
b. The slope of the characteristic curve depends upon development processes.
c. Subject x-ray contrast depends on the differential attenuation of the x-ray beam as it passes through the patient.
d. Radiographic contrast is the product of subjective (perceived) contrast and film contrast.
e. If the average gradient of the film is greater than 1, the subject contrast of the film will be decreased.

4.19 Film contrast is influenced by:

a. The concentration of the developer used.
b. Presence or absence of an intensifying screen.
c. The type of emulsion used.
d. Time of development.
e. The level of base plus fog.

4.20 Radiographic contrast may be increased by:

a. Reducing scattered radiation.
b. Using a film with a high gamma.
c. Applying compression to the body part.
d. Using an x-ray anti-scatter grid.
e. Increasing the thickness of the x-ray beam filtration.

4.21 Radiographic contrast is affected by:

a. Limitation of field size.
b. Incorrect development conditions.
c. Oxidation of developing agents.
d. Variations in the electron density of the tissue.
e. Atomic number of the structures of the subject.

4.22 Rare earths:

a. Rare earth elements are relatively abundant.
b. Rare earth screens have a lower conversion efficiency from x-ray energy to light photons when compared to a calcium tungstate screen.
c. Rare earths typically have an x-ray K absorption edge below 70 kV.
d. Rare earth elements used in intensifying screens include gadolinium, yttrium and lanthanum.
e. Rare earth screens may emit blue light.

4.23 Intensifying screens for medical radiography are commonly produced using the following phosphors:

a. Lanthanum oxybromide.
b. Zinc cadmium sulphide.
c. Sodium iodide (activated with thallium).
d. Barium lead sulphate.
e. Gadolinium oxysulphide (activated with terbium).

4.24 The speed of a film–screen system:

a. Is the exposure needed to produce unit density above base plus fog.
b. Is increased by increased phosphor crystal grain size.
c. Is increased by raising the temperature of the developer.
d. Is increased by lengthening the time of development.
e. Is independent of the shape of the silver halide crystals.

4.25 Concerning intensifying screens:

a. They function by emitting electrons when bombarded with x-rays.
b. They reduce the effect of film grain size.
c. Shorter exposures are possible, reducing the risk of movement blur.
d. Screen–film contact can be tested by using a perforated metal plate or mesh.
e. Repeated x-ray exposures eventually lead to screen failure.

4.26 Regarding the intensification factor (IF):

a. The intensification factor is the ratio of *exposure needed to produce an image with film alone* and to *exposure needed for film and screen.*
b. The intensification factor is of no relevance to patient dose.
c. Increasing the IF of the film–screen combination will result in a higher dose to the patient.
d. It may be increased by making the phosphor layer thicker.
e. It may be increased by the introduction of a layer of titanium dioxide between the base and the phosphor layer.

4.27 Regarding intensifying screens:

a. Screen efficiency describes the ability of a screen to absorb and convert x-ray photon energy into light.
b. Increasing the intrinsic conversion efficiency of a screen improves the noise.
c. Increasing the screen thickness increases the noise.
d. The presence of a reflective layer increases the noise.
e. Increasing the x-ray absorption efficiency of a screen results in a noisier image.

4.28 Quality control information that can be derived from a sensitometric test strip includes:

a. Spatial resolution.
b. Optical density as a result of exposure.
c. Contrast index.
d. Base plus fog.
e. Relative film speed.

4.29　Single emulsion film is usually used for:

a. Extremity radiography.
b. Mammography.
c. Nuclear medicine.
d. Dental radiographs.
e. Laser hardcopy film.

4.30　Anti-scatter grids:

a. Are usually made of lead strips with copper between them.
b. With a focused grid, film focus distance is relatively fixed.
c. Can be placed on both sides of patient.
d. If focused the grid must be focused onto the patient.
e. A non-focused grid can be reversed for use.

4.31　Regarding the use of an anti-scatter grid:

a. Dose to the patient is increased.
b. It causes a deterioration in the contrast of an image.
c. Lateral decentring of a grid gives a lighter film.
d. Using the incorrect film focus distance with a focused grid leads to uniformly dark film.
e. High ratio grids are used in low kV techniques.

4.32　Doubling the focus film distance (FFD) for the same photographic density, and keeping all other factors, including the object–film distance, equal:

a. Requires increasing the exposure by a factor of two.
b. Decreases the area of skin irradiated at the entrance surface, if collimation is not changed.
c. Increases the entrance surface dose.
d. Produces a large change in the volume of tissue irradiated.
e. Requires a more penetrating x-ray beam to be employed.

4.1 Answers

a. True – this attracts stray electrons in close proximity to the envelope. Because of its low atomic number, any electrons interacting with it will produce only low energy radiation, which is easily absorbed in the tube housing.

b. False – although these photons are often of lower energy than those produced at the focal spot, they are energetic enough to contribute to patient dose and to degrade image quality.

c. False – the opposite is true.

d. False – it increases geometric unsharpness and reduces subject x-ray contrast.

e. True – some of the extrafocal radiation is produced in this way.

4.2 Answers

a. True – a smaller angle produces a foreshortened effective focal spot when compared with the true focal spot size.

b. True – the smaller the electron beam hitting the target, the smaller the resultant focal spot.

c. False – it depends on the size of the electron beam striking the target, and on the anode angle. This does not depend on the physical size of the anode.

d. False – see c.

e. True – due to foreshortening by the anode angle.

4.3 Answers

a. True – using a pinhole much smaller (0.03 mm) than the focal spot size (0.3–1 mm) the effective focal spot size can be estimated. A Star Test Pattern can be used to obtain similar information.

b. False – the target angle is the angle between the target and the axial x-ray. A smaller target angle decreases effective focal spot size by foreshortening the focal spot as seen from a point on the axial ray.

c. False – at very high tube currents the electron beam diverges because of repulsion of individual electrons by negative charge, a process known as blooming. This may be noticeable when a low kV is used leading to an increase in focal spot size of up to 10%.

d. False – the electron beam increases in size by 10% at low kV. This is caused by an increase in the space charge effect and will increase the effective focal spot size.

e. False – this only affects the rating of the tube.

4.4 Answers

a. **False** – this would limit movement unsharpness.
b. **False** – it improves unsharpness by reducing geometric unsharpness.
c. **True** – screen unsharpness is caused by light diffusion in the screen itself, which reduces resolution.
d. **True** – film unsharpness is caused by crossover of light between the two layers, and by parallax when viewing the image.
e. **False** – the size of the penumbra around the image will be limited by a short object–film distance, and this will reduce geometric unsharpness.

4.5 Answers

a. **True** – at a large focus–object distance, the apparent size of the focal spot is smaller, and it more closely approximates to a point source. This reduces the penumbra formed and results in less geometric unsharpness.
b. **True** – with low subject contrast, noise limits resolution. For this reason high contrast test objects are used to measure spatial resolution.
c. **True** – a high output tube will allow high currents and shorter exposure times as a result. This may help to limit movement unsharpness.
d. **False** – it will reduce scatter which may otherwise degrade the radiographic contrast but will not improve spatial resolution.
e. **False** – increasing kV reduces subject contrast and narrows the grey scale available for image formation. This will make the detection of small differences in tissue density more difficult on a radiograph.

4.6 Answers

a. **True** – geometric blur depends on two factors: focal spot size and geometric magnification. Reducing either will reduce the size of any penumbra.
b. **False** – this produces edge unsharpness, which is caused when an object's thickness tapers towards its edge. The optical density of its image fades gradually from high to low, and the actual position of the edge may be hard to define. It is not related to geometric unsharpness.
c. **False** – this will influence movement unsharpness by affecting the exposure time.
d. **True** – this will change the geometric magnification – see a.
e. **False** – this may affect movement unsharpness by changing the exposure time, and the reduced contrast may also affect the edge unsharpness or the ability to perceive small fine detail, but the size of the penumbra will not be changed.

4.7 Answers

a. **False** – a pinhole can measure focal spot size, which is related to resolution, but it will not measure resolution itself. A line pair test object is used for this purpose.

b. **True** – increasing the geometric magnification requires either a smaller focus–object distance or a larger object–film distance. Either of these changes will increase the size of the penumbra.

c. **True** – this may then be used for comparison of different imaging systems.

d. **False** – spatial resolution is comparable in modern computed radiography.

e. **True** – and by the number of lines on the monitor. These two factors determine the pixel size.

4.8 Answers

a. **True** – the formal definition is the magnitude of the Fourier transformed line spread function. It is used to assess the overall spatial resolution of an imaging system.

b. **True** – the MTF is derived from the line spread function using a one-dimensional Fourier transformation and is proportional to the ratio of the signal information recorded to the signal information potentially available (i.e. a measure of information loss in the image compared with the object).

c. **True** – by definition MTF is independent of mottle because exposure settings are optimised to remove its effect from the image.

d. **False** – see a.

e. **False** – a system cannot resolve at a spatial frequency where the MTF is zero, though a practical limit may be defined as an MTF of less than 0.1. An MTF of one indicates perfect reproduction of the signal.

4.9 Answers

a. **False** – it is the product of these values.

b. **False** – in film–screen radiography the maximum value is 1.0. However in digital image enhancement the MTF can be greater than this because of edge enhancement improving spatial resolution.

c. **True** – the maximum resolution in a mammography system is 20 line pairs (lp)/mm compared to 10 lp mm^{-1} for a high definition system.

d. **True** – non-screen film can resolve 100 lp mm^{-1}. An intensifying screen reduces this to 5–10 lp mm^{-1}, because of its poorer MTF.

e. **True** – and the size of the pixels sampled.

4.10 Answers

a. **False** – it decreases.

b. **False** – the reverse is true, because of the effect of increasing geometric unsharpness.

c. **True** – primarily the number of pixels limits the resolution in the image. If the image is magnified, it is distributed over more pixels, allowing smaller detail to be resolved. In principle, the resolution could be improved by magnification until further improvement is limited by the unsharpness of the image on the input phosphor of the intensifier.

d. **False** – the MTF of the film–screen combination is by definition independent of the effects of other components of the imaging system, i.e. focal spot size will not have any bearing on its measurement.

e. **False** – a gamma camera can typically resolve a maximum of 1 line pair per centimetre. There are two ways to produce a measurement. The camera could image two point sources of radioactivity with varying degrees of separation or a line source could be used and the line spread function measured.

4.11 Answers

a. **True** – anti-scatter grids selectively 'filter out' scatter from the beam emerging from the patient. Both focused and unfocused grids do this.

b. **False** – with a large field more scatter is generated.

c. **False** – scatter photons exiting the patient at wide angles are more likely to bypass the image receptor than undeflected primary photons if an air gap technique, with a larger object–film distance, is used.

d. **False** – this has no effect. However, using a longer focus-film distance may allow an air gap technique to be used with only a small increase in patient dose.

e. **False** – this only limits movement unsharpness.

4.12 Answers

a. **False** – if this occurs, then either the dose will be higher, and the proportion of scatter will stay the same, or the field size will be greater, which will increase scatter production.

b. **True** – compression reduces the thickness, but not the density, of tissue in the beam, because tissue is pushed out of the way. This will reduce attenuation within the patient, so that less radiation is required and there will be fewer scattering events. The proportion of scatter to transmitted radiation will decrease as a consequence.

c. **True** – this makes secondary (scattered) radiation less penetrating and less likely to reach the film.

d. **False** – this will not reduce scatter.

e. **True** – scatter from the back surface of the cassette is minimised if the back is made from a high atomic number material, which will absorb rather than scatter the photons.

4.13 Answers

a. **False** – because of quality control in intensifying screen production, structure mottle makes a negligible contribution to total noise relative to the quantum mottle from the high speed of the screen.

b. **False** – this has no effect on mottle, but will help to reduce the necessary exposure and therefore the patient dose.

c. **True**.

d. **False** – with geometric magnification the level of quantum noise remains constant while the size of the image signal increases. This leads to an improvement in the signal to noise ratio. When the image is then reduced in size by optical demagnification, the level of recorded noise is suppressed in the final image.

e. **True** – by amplifying the low intensity noise signal in the image.

4.14 Answers

a. **False** – this will reduce the effect of quantum mottle.

b. **False** – this would produce structure mottle.

c. **True** – see a.

d. **False** – generally, heat rating has nothing to do with noise, though a tube with a low heat rating may not be able to produce a high enough output to expose the film adequately.

e. **True** – at high kV fewer photons are required to form the image because the speed of the system increases at higher kV.

4.15 Answers

a. **False** – a subdued level of ambient lighting is required.

b. **False** – uncovered parts of the illuminator degrade visual perception. It is more difficult to differentiate subtle shades of grey when next to bright light.

c. **False** – they should be matched to allow comparison.

d. **False** – radiographic contrast is the product of subject x-ray contrast and film contrast, and therefore is independent of subjective parameters. Subjective (or perceived) contrast relies on the perception of the viewer, and is dependent on viewing conditions.

e. **False** – it responds in a logarithmic manner.

4.16 Answers

a. **True** – current theories of latent image formation are based on this description, proposed in 1938.
b. **False** – one photon of light is sufficient for one electron to migrate to the sensitivity spot. On average five or more light photons per grain are required for a developable latent image.
c. **True** – when a photon of light of energy greater than a certain minimum value is absorbed in a silver bromide crystal, an electron is released from a bromide ion. The electron is free to move about the crystal. When it reaches a latent image site, it may be 'trapped' there, giving the latent image site a negative electrical charge. The latent image site is also known as the sensitivity speck.
d. **True** – the negatively charged trap can then attract a positive interstitial silver ion. When such an interstitial ion reaches a negatively charged trap, its charge is neutralised and an atom of silver is deposited at the trap.
e. **True** – this whole cycle can recur many times at a single trap, each cycle involving absorption of one photon and addition of one silver atom. This aggregate of silver atoms is the latent image. The presence of these few atoms at the latent image site makes the whole grain susceptible to the reducing action of the developer.

4.17 Answers

a. **False** – it is a graph of optical density as a function of log to the base ten (or $\log_{10}$) of the exposure.
b. **True**.
c. **True** – film contrast is a measure of how the film responds to subject x-ray contrast. It depends on four main factors: the characteristic curve of the film (i.e. gamma), film density, screen or direct x-ray exposure and the film processing.
d. **False** – they are inversely proportional. A film with a high gamma has a steep gradient curve, and so a narrow latitude.
e. **True**.

4.18 Answers

a. **True**.
b. **True** – development processes influence film contrast.
c. **True** – this depends on the tissue thickness, density, kVp, contrast media and scatter radiation.
d. **False** – it is the product of subject x-ray contrast and film contrast. Consequently anything that affects either of these two parameters will alter radiographic contrast.
e. **False** – the radiographic contrast will be emphasised.

4.19 Answers

a. **True** – the type, activity and degree of agitation of the developer affects the film gamma.
b. **True** – the gamma of the film will be greatest when the film is exposed with intensifying screens.
c. **True** – uniformity of the distribution of crystal sizes within the emulsion affects gamma.
d. **True** – increasing the development time will initially increase film gamma, then decrease it. The same pattern is seen with increased temperature of development.
e. **True** – an elevated base plus fog level will lower the average gradient.

4.20 Answers

a. **True** – scattered radiation decreases image contrast.
b. **True** – as this determines film contrast.
c. **True** – decreasing thickness decreases the proportion of x-ray scatter produced.
d. **True** – x-ray contrast is improved by reducing scattered x-rays.
e. **False** – an x-ray beam filter increases the mean energy of the x-ray beam, making it more penetrative. This reduces subject x-ray contrast.

4.21 Answers

a. **True** – by reducing x-ray scatter, contrast is improved, demonstrating the importance of collimation.
b. **True** – incorrect temperature, replenishment rates, chemical mixing or film fogging all decrease film contrast.
c. **True** – as the film contrast will be decreased.
d. **True** – as the electron density of the material affects the attenuation of x-rays, and hence the subject contrast.
e. **True** – as atomic number will affect the degree of attenuation, and therefore the subject contrast.

4.22 Answers

a. **True** – despite the misnomer rare earths! They are called 'rare' because they are difficult to isolate and expensive to extract.
b. **False** – better conversion (15% compared with 5%).
c. **True** – K absorption edge of gadolinium is 50 keV, tungsten is at 70 keV.
d. **True**.
e. **True** – e.g. lanthanum oxybromide activated with terbium. Other rare earth phosphors such as gadolinium oxysuplide activated with terbium emit green light.

4.23 Answers

a. **True**.
b. **False** – output phosphor in image intensifier.
c. **False** – this is the phosphor crystal used in the gamma camera.
d. **False** – no longer used.
e. **True**.

4.24 Answers

a. **False** – it may be defined as the reciprocal of the exposure that produces unit density above base plus fog.
b. **True** – compared with smaller grains, larger grains will intercept more photons but will only require the same number of interactions to become developable.
c. **True** – see d.
d. **True** – increasing the time of development increases the number of chemical reactions, and therefore the speed. The same effect is achieved by increasing the temperature of developer.
e. **False** – flat (tabular) crystals that are aligned to the x-ray beam produce a faster film than rounder crystals.

4.25 Answers

a. **False** – they absorb x-ray photons and emit light of an intensity proportional to that of the incident x-ray beam.
b. **True** – film graininess is reduced due to light diffusion in the phosphor layer.
c. **True** – this is one of the benefits of a fast imaging system.
d. **True** – the plate or mesh is placed on the cassette and exposed. Any areas that are poorly defined will correspond to areas of poor film–screen contact.
e. **False** – failure is mechanical through wear, not excessive irradiation.

4.26 Answers

a. **True** – typical values are 30–100.
b. **False** – the greater the intensification factor, the lower is the dose needed to produce the desired optical density.
c. **False** – a greater intensification factor implies a faster system and less dose, although image quality may deteriorate.
d. **True** – this increases x-ray photon absorption efficiency.
e. **True** – this is a reflective layer, and reflects any light that is travelling away from the film which would otherwise be lost.

4.27 Answers

a. **True** – screen efficiency is the combination of x-ray absorption efficiency, that is the ability of the screen to absorb x-ray photons, and intrinsic conversion efficiency, which is the ability of the screen to convert x-ray photons into light photons.

b. **False** – there is more noise as fewer light photons are absorbed for the same photographic density. Speed increases but spatial resolution is unaffected.

c. **False** – the noise remains the same as the same numbers of x-ray photons will be absorbed for the same film density. The thicker screen will increase speed but produce poorer spatial resolution.

d. **True** – a reflective layer reduces the number of x-ray photons that are needed for the same optical density, thus increasing noise and speed, but decreasing the spatial resolution.

e. **False** – the exposure for the same film blackening is reduced and therefore speed increases, but if the same number of x-ray photons have been absorbed, the noise and resolution will be the same.

4.28 Answers

a. **False** – this is obtained using a resolution test grating.

b. **True** – this can be measured using a calibrated optical densitometer.

c. **True** – this is the optical density difference between specified densities.

d. **True** – this is the optical density of the unexposed part of the film.

e. **True** – this can be derived from the film at the point where the optical density is unity above the base plus fog.

4.29 Answers

a. **True** – with anti-halation backing to prevent light reflection, for high definition.

b. **True** – single emulsion is used to reduce parallax and ensure optimal spatial resolution.

c. **True** – single-sided transparency film is used because only visible light is being recorded.

d. **False** – double emulsion films are required to increase x-ray absorption (no intensifying screens are used).

e. **True**.

4.30 Answers

a. **False** – interspaces are made of radiolucent material.
b. **True** – if the small focusing range is exceeded, grid cut off may occur.
c. **False** – their purpose is to absorb scatter in the beam exiting the patient, so they must only be used on the film side.
d. **False** – the paths of x-rays traversing the grid converge at the x-ray focal spot.
e. **True** – with no loss of primary radiation. However, a focused grid must be correctly oriented.

4.31 Answers

a. **True** – a parallel grid will remove up to 30% of primary (unscattered) x-ray photons. The x-ray tube output must therefore be increased as a result to allow adequate film exposure.
b. **False** – by the removal of up to 90% of scatter radiation, the contrast of the image will be improved. This is known as the contrast improvement factor of a grid, and is normally between 2 and 4.
c. **True** – this increases as the amount of decentring increases.
d. **False** – the film will be of a lower optical density towards the periphery of the grid.
e. **False** – they are only used in high kV techniques.

4.32 Answers

a. **False** – the inverse square law states that the intensity of an x-ray beam will decrease as the inverse of the square of the distance from the x-ray source. Absorption of the x-ray beam in the patient will be the same, so only the effect of the increased FFD need be considered. If the distance is doubled then the exposure has to increase by a factor of 4 to achieve the same film blackening.
b. **False** – the rays are diverging so a larger area of the skin would be irradiated, although normally the beam would be collimated to keep the area the same.
c. **False** – both the FFD and the focus–skin distance (FSD) are increased. Since the FSD is, by definition, less than the FFD, it is increased by a greater fraction, so the reduction in dose (due to the inverse square law) at the FSD is greater than at the FFD. Therefore the reduction in dose at the FSD more than makes up for the increase in exposure needed to keep the optical density the same.
d. **False** – if the field size at the patient is kept constant, the volume will decrease slightly. If the field size at the film is kept constant, the volume will increase slightly. Either way, the change will be small.
e. **False** – the same film blackening is achieved, so the same kV could be used if the mAs is increased appropriately.

5. Conventional film processing

5.1   Regarding photographic density:

   a. It is a quantitative measurement of the blackening of a film after exposure and processing.

   b. The term photographic density is defined as the logarithm to the base 10 (or $\log_{10}$) of the opacity.

   c. Transmittence is defined as the ratio of the intensity of transmitted light to the intensity of light incident on the film.

   d. A photographic density of 2.0 reduces light intensity by a factor of 100.

   e. A film with a photographic density of 2.0 transmits half as much light as a film with a photographic density of 1.0.

5.2   Regarding film faults:

   a. Opaque, high density marks on a film may be caused by fixer splashed on the unexposed film.

   b. An incompletely fixed film will be brown.

   c. Static marks may cause white marks on the film.

   d. Crease and pressure marks may be seen if films are stored and handled inappropriately.

   e. Film faults may occur if the developer temperature is too low.

5.3   Base plus fog is:

   a. The optical density of the film base, plus that of the unexposed emulsion.

   b. Partially caused by the development of unexposed silver halide grains.

   c. Increased by a high level of humidity during storage.

   d. Increased by using a more sensitive film.

   e. Affected by background radiation.

5.4   Base plus fog:

   a. Is increased by pressure on the films during storage.

   b. Is affected by the temperature of the developer.

   c. Is increased by the use of a moving grid rather than a fixed grid.

   d. Is decreased by additives such as potassium bromide.

   e. Is increased if too bright a safelight is used.

5.5　In development of an x-ray film:

a. The developer is a reducing agent (electron donor).
b. Development is affected by reduction of the developing agents.
c. The developer contains alkali as a decelerator.
d. Developing agents also reduce unexposed silver halide crystals, but at a lower rate.
e. Phenidone/hydroquinone is an example of developer chemistry.

5.1 Answers

a. True.

b. True – where the opacity is defined as the ratio of light incident to that transmitted by the film. Photographic density is also known as optical density and film density.

c. True – on this basis the term opacity is the reciprocal of transmission.

d. True – as $\log_{10} 100 = 2$, the ratio of incident to transmitted light is $100 : 1$. In simple terms, for every 100 photons incident on the film, only one photon, or 1% (0.01) is transmitted.

e. False – a photographic density of 1.0 equates to 10% light transmission and a density of 2.0 equates to 1% transmission. Therefore a film with a photographic density of 2.0 will transmit one tenth of the light that a film with a photographic density of 1.0 will transmit.

5.2 Answers

a. True.

b. False – the fixer prevents further development by removing the unexposed silver grains. The film would appear milky, because small silver crystals would not be dissolved and washed away.

c. False – static marks are black marks on the film, caused by electrostatic discharge due to low humidity in the air or films being pulled out of the packet too quickly.

d. True – especially if films are stored horizontal not vertically. They appear as an opaque mark causing distortion of the image.

e. True – this would result in a film with insufficient blackening.

5.3 Answers

a. True – the base density is due to the intrinsic film base density. Film fog is caused by the development of unexposed silver halide grains. Together these give a base plus fog density of between 0.1 and 0.2, depending on the film type and processing conditions.

b. True – if the development time is too long then this will increase the development of unexposed silver halide grains, which increases film fog.

c. True – increased humidity and temperature increases fog.

d. True – sensitive films form latent images more easily (e.g. during development).

e. True – exposure to high amounts of extraneous radiation will cause fogging.

5.4 Answers

a. True – films should be stored vertically on their sides, not piled on top of each other.
b. True – higher developer temperatures increase fog.
c. False – although both reduce contrast they have no effect on fog.
d. True – anti-foggants are added during development.
e. True – film fog is increased in this way, or if the safelight is the wrong colour or is positioned too close to the film handling area.

5.5 Answers

a. True – the developer reduces exposed silver bromide to metallic silver.
b. False – oxidation of developer shortens its life. Preservatives (e.g. sodium sulphite) are added to the developer to minimise oxidation and its effects.
c. False – this acts as an accelerator. Most developers have a pH 10–11.5.
d. True – this explains why timing of development is crucial. The addition of a restrainer, typically potassium bromide, helps the unexposed silver bromide crystals to maintain a barrier of bromide ions around them, thus preventing reduction and fog formation.
e. True – these act synergistically, another example is metol/hydroquinone.

6. Quality assurance and quality control

6.1   **Regarding measurements normally used in quality assurance testing:**

    a. A potential divider is normally used to measure kVp.
    b. A densitometer can be used to measure film density and calculate gamma.
    c. An acceptable error in the predicted kV is ±5 kV.
    d. An acceptable error in the x-ray beam alignment is 10% compared with the light beam.
    e. It is permitted for the measured focal spot size to be larger than the specified tube value by up to 50%.

6.2   **Quality assurance on equipment should:**

    a. Be undertaken to ensure the continual production of optimum quality images with the minimum necessary dose to the patient.
    b. Result in a reduction of radiation dose to radiographers.
    c. Be carried out to enable compliance with IRR 1999.
    d. Audit any films that are deemed of an unacceptable quality.
    e. Include acceptance testing prior to any equipment being introduced to clinical use.

6.1 Answers

a. **False** – an electronic penetrameter is normally used to measure the penetration of x-rays when placed in the primary beam from an x-ray tube and estimates the kVp from this. A potential divider is an invasive kV measurement device that is not normally used for quality assurance (QA) checks.

b. **True** – after a series of exposures a film test strip can be analysed with a densitometer and a characteristic film curve can be plotted. This can then be used to calculate film gamma.

c. **True** – for conventional x-ray work, this is regarded as an acceptable tolerance. In mammography, the tube voltage is expected to be correct to within ±1 kV.

d. **True** – each edge of the x-ray field should be within 1 cm of the edge of the light field for a 20×20 field at 1 m. This means an error of up to 10% is possible.

e. **True** – 25–50% variation is allowed from the manufacturer's specification.

6.2 Answers

a. **True**.

b. **True** – if patient doses are reduced, there will be a consequent reduction in scattered radiation in the x-ray room. Also, the QA checks may reveal faults such as excessive radiation leakage from the x-ray machine.

c. **True** – QA is a requirement of the regulations and a record of the testing and the maintenance record should be kept for each item of x-ray equipment.

d. **True** – this may enable the number of repeated radiographs to be reduced.

e. **True** – to ensure that it performs to specification and operates safely.

7. Mammography

7.1 Regarding mammography:

a. Compression can be used to reduce the patient dose.
b. The maximum compression permitted for a breast is a force of 200 N.
c. It is a low dose technique and carries a negligible cancer risk in all women.
d. A focus to film distance of at least 100 cm is used.
e. The mean glandular dose to the breast must be less than 2 mGy.

7.2 In mammography:

a. A K edge filter may be used.
b. A rhodium target used instead of molybdenum will produce an x-ray beam with a higher mean energy.
c. The grid moves continuously during the exposure.
d. Failure of the Reciprocity Law may result in poorer image quality.
e. Boron is normally chosen as the tube window because of its low attenuation properties.

7.3 In a mammographic x-ray tube:

a. There may be more than one target track on the anode.
b. The tube voltage is typically 35–40 kV.
c. The axial ray is directed to the centre of the x-ray field.
d. The anode does not rotate.
e. The focal spot size is typically 0.5 mm.

7.4 The following are true of radiograph production and viewing for a mammogram:

a. Dual emulsion films are used to improve image contrast.
b. The intensifying screen is placed behind the film.
c. A low gamma film is used.
d. A high exposure latitude is required of the film.
e. The optimum film density for viewing is 1.5–2.0.

7.5   **In mammography:**

a. To image a thick breast a target anode combination using molybdenum–molybdenum is the most appropriate.
b. If a molybdenum anode is filtered by a molybdenum target, only high energy photons are removed from the beam.
c. Breast compression is not important because of the short exposure times used.
d. Rare earth screens are used.
e. As breast thickness increases contrast is reduced.

7.6   **In mammography:**

a. The x-ray photon energy range is selected to allow photoelectric effects to predominate over scatter.
b. Grids are not used because of increased dose to the breast.
c. Tungsten targets are not used because of the lack of characteristic radiation produced at low kV.
d. At low kV, x-ray output is approximately proportional to the kV cubed.
e. Subject contrast is important whereas geometric unsharpness is not.

7.1 Answers

a. **True** – a lower exposure is required with reduced breast thickness, which results in a lower dose. However, the main purpose of compression is to improve image quality.

b. **True** – equivalent to about 20 kgf (kilogram force).

c. **False** – although the dose is relatively low, the risk of cancer induction is sufficient to be a factor in determining the optimum age range of the population selected for a screening programme.

d. **False** – 60 cm is common. The low kV, small focal spot and relatively low amount of bremsstrahlung produced creates a relatively low output system. A larger FFD would result in problems with achieving sufficiently high exposures.

e. **False** – this was a limit applied in the UK breast-screening programme for a 'standard breast'. Larger breasts might well require greater doses. The diagnostic reference level for the breast screening programme has been set at a mean glandular dose of 3.5 mGy for a 55 mm thick compressed breast.

7.2 Answers

a. **True** – e.g. rhodium in conjunction with a rhodium or tungsten target, or more commonly, a molybdenum filter with a molybdenum target.

b. **True** – characteristic x-rays dominate the spectrum from a mammographic x-ray set. Characteristic radiation from rhodium has higher energy peaks at 20.2 and 22.8 keV compared with 17.8 and 19.7 keV from a molybdenum target.

c. **True** – this ensures the grid lines are blurred out of the radiograph.

d. **True** – if the exposure time to deliver a set tube output (mAs) is long (i.e. with a low mA setting) then latent image centres formed in film by light photons from the screen can revert to their normal state before the grain is developed. In other words the degree of film blackening will not be proportional to the exposure (mAs). This is failure of the Reciprocity Law.

e. **False** – a beryllium window is used for this purpose.

7.3 Answers

a. True – modern tubes allow selection of both the filter and the target. For example a Mo target with either a Mo or Rh filter, or Rh or W target with a Rh filter.
b. False – the usual range is 25–30 kV.
c. False – the anode heel effect is utilised in mammography to allow the more intense part of the beam to be directed at the thickest part of the breast. The axial ray is therefore directed at the chest wall and the anode side of the beam is not used. The axial ray is the ray produced from the centre of the focal spot.
d. False – the small focal spot and long exposures required in mammography place significant heating loads on the tube. A rotating anode is therefore essential to improve the heat rating.
e. False – general mammograms require a 0.3 mm focal spot and a 0.1 mm spot for magnification work to limit geometric unsharpness.

7.4 Answers

a. False – a single emulsion film is used to reduce film unsharpness due to the parallax effect in image recording on double emulsion film.
b. True – because the photons are of low energy, they are absorbed strongly near the entrance surface of the screen. Placing the film in front of the screen reduces the distance light must travel through the screen to reach the film and minimises the light absorption by the screen itself. A vacuum cassette is often used to ensure good film–screen contact to facilitate this.
c. False – a high gamma film (greater than 3) is needed for adequate contrast because subject contrast is low.
d. False – gamma and latitude are inversely related. Films therefore have low latitude as a result of the requirement for high contrast.
e. True – assuming ambient viewing conditions are optimised.

7.5 Answers

a. False – a molybdenum–rhodium or rhodium–rhodium combination would produce an x-ray beam with a higher mean energy than molybdenum–molybdenum. This makes the beam more able to penetrate the thicker breast.
b. False – the filter strongly absorbs radiation with energy above the K edge of molybdenum, while being relatively transparent to the characteristic radiation peaks (17.5 keV and 19.6 keV), but it also absorbs low energy photons. It therefore removes both high and low energy photons, and transmits those with the optimum energy for good image contrast.
c. False – as well as reducing dose, compression reduces movement unsharpness. Relatively long exposures are required to produce enough film blackening at such a low kV without exceeding the tube rating.
d. True – to reduce patient dose and optimise image quality.
e. True – due to the increased amount of scatter.

7.6 Answers

a. **True** – the optimum photon energy for this is around 20 keV.

b. **False** – high image quality requires a high resolution moving grid. This increases glandular dose by a factor of between 2 and 3. A standard grid ratio for mammography is 4–5.

c. **False** – the bremsstrahlung spectrum can be modified by using a rhodium K edge filter (K edge 23.3 keV) to remove high energy photons. However, molybdenum or rhodium targets are more commonly used, as they produce a more effective spectrum of energies for breast imaging.

d. **True** – in contrast with general radiography with higher kV, where the relationship is proportional to kV squared.

e. **False** – the balance of both factors is important. Hence the desire for low kV technique and compression with high gamma film–screen combinations and as small a focal spot as possible.

8. Special radiographic techniques

8.1 The high kilovoltage technique for chest radiography:

a. Results in increased radiographic contrast.
b. Gives greater exposure latitude.
c. Increases the quantity of scattered radiation reaching the film.
d. A grid is mandatory.
e. If a grid is used, a ratio of 5 : 1 would be appropriate.

8.2 Use of the high kV technique (100 kV and over):

a. Results in an increased radiation dose to the patient for the same film blackening.
b. Shows better bone detail.
c. Cardiac movement blurring is decreased.
d. The detail at the hilar regions on a PA chest x-ray is improved.
e. Obviates the need for filtration of the x-ray beam.

8.3 In tomography:

a. Short exposures are essential.
b. The thickness of cut decreases with increased angle of swing.
c. Zonography typically uses 30–50° angles of arc.
d. Phantom image formation is less of a problem in zonography.
e. Blur margins are not a problem in linear tomography.

8.4 Regarding tomography:

a. The technique is no longer practised in modern departments.
b. Wide angle tomograms produce optimal images of high contrast structures.
c. The focal plane is centred on the position of the fulcrum.
d. Focal plane images are sharper in zonography.
e. The tube and film cassette move independently of each other.

8.5 Macroradiography:

a. Results in a minified image.
b. Requires longer exposure times when compared to general radiography.
c. A grid is essential to improve image unsharpness.
d. Uses a focal spot less than 0.3 mm in size.
e. The technique involves higher entrance surface doses of radiation to the patient.

8.6 Regarding paediatric imaging:

a. The risk from the radiation is greater than for adults.
b. Exposure times should be longer.
c. A grid must be used.
d. Added filters are mandatory.
e. The risk of cancer induction before the age of 15 is about 6% per sievert.

8.1 Answers

a. **False** – decreased radiographic contrast.
b. **True** – subject x-ray contrast is reduced, allowing a wider range of anatomical detail to be recorded by the film.
c. **True** – up to five times more scatter reaches the film.
d. **False** – an air gap is just as efficient and results in less dose to the patient.
e. **False** – 10 : 1 is a good choice and gives comparable contrast to a 20 cm air gap.

8.2 Answers

a. **False** – the more penetrative beam allows a reduced mAs setting to be used, so the entrance surface dose is marginally less.
b. **False** – rib detail is lost as there is lower subject contrast at higher kV.
c. **True** – because of the shorter exposure, movement due to respiration and cardiac movement is decreased.
d. **True** – due to the reduction in contrast the definition between the hila and lungs is less, but the detail within soft tissues is better depicted due to the wider grey scale that is available.
e. **False** – the x-ray beam still needs filtration.

8.3 Answers

a. **False** – a continuous exposure or series of shorter exposure are required for the duration of movement of the tube for wide angles of swing. In short angle tomography relatively short exposures are possible, but longer than for a standard radiograph.
b. **True** – wide angle tomograms produce thin slices and vice versa.
c. **False** – also called narrow angle tomography, a 5–10° arc is used to take a thick cut.
d. **False** – this is one of the main drawbacks of this technique and is caused by structures outside the focal plane overlapping to produce an apparent image which does not represent a real structure. This is much less of a problem with wide angles of arc.
e. **False** – blur is a significant problem in linear tomograms and worsens with increasing angles of swing. This is caused by constant variation in the distance of the x-ray tube and film from the subject (e.g. the kidney) during an exposure, which results in distortion of the final image. More complex tomographic movements tend to mirror the shape of anatomical structures (e.g. circular, elliptic) and reduce this effect.

8.4 Answers

a. **False** – intravenous urograms and assessment of bone fracture union in complex cases are the main uses of this technique. Tomography of other body parts has been superseded by computed tomography.

b. **True** – such as bone. Zonography is better at demonstrating low contrast soft tissue structures, e.g. lungs and kidneys.

c. **True** – the region of interest must be positioned at the level of the fulcrum, as this is the point in the image that remains in focus while the rest of the image blurs.

d. **True** – this is the main advantage of the technique as greater arcs of movement reduce image sharpness. This allows low contrast structures to be visualised.

e. **False** – it is essential that their movement is coordinated precisely. For this reason they are attached by a rigid rod that rotates about the fulcrum.

8.5 Answers

a. **False** – a magnified image is produced because the focus–object distance is decreased relative to the object–film distance.

b. **True** – in general longer exposure times are needed, so immobilisation is important to minimise movement unsharpness.

c. **False** – the air gap obviates the need for a grid.

d. **True** – magnification increases geometric unsharpness, so to retain high detail resolution, a smaller focal spot size is needed, for example a 0.1 mm focal spot for imaging microcalcifications in mammography.

e. **True** – as an increased exposure is needed and the patient is closer to the focal spot.

8.6 Answers

a. **True** – the risk is greater to lower age groups, and children have a longer life expectancy within which to express radiation damage.

b. **False** – children may be less able to follow instructions for keeping still and holding their breath, so shorter times are desirable to minimise movement unsharpness.

c. **False** – less scatter is produced so the increased dose is not normally warranted.

d. **False** – added filters may be used in fluoroscopy to force the automatic brightness control to increase the kV, which reduces the dose. However they are not a requirement.

e. **False** – this would be true for irradiation in utero, but not for children in general. This would certainly not apply to a 14 year old child.

9. Image intensifiers and fluoroscopy

9.1   **In the image intensifier:**

a. For a 25 cm diameter image intensifier, the output phosphor is typically 2.5 cm in diameter.
b. Zinc cadmium sulphide activated with silver is used as the output phosphor.
c. Sodium activated caesium iodide is chosen as the input phosphor because a thick crystal layer can be formed with minimum loss of spatial resolution.
d. The photocathode converts incident high speed electrons into light.
e. The TV monitor gives a similar spatial resolution to that available from a film–screen system.

9.2   **In a fluoroscopic examination:**

a. Patient dose rates are commonly in the range 10–20 mGy per second.
b. The skin dose rate may be 300 times greater than the image intensifier input dose rates.
c. The quantum sink in image formation is the input phosphor screen.
d. Electrodes are used to focus and minify the electron image.
e. In an image intensifier, a single x-ray photon at the input screen causes about 500–1000 light photons to be emitted from the output screen.

9.3   **When using image intensifiers in fluoroscopy:**

a. The maximum fluoroscopy current is limited by the focal spot size.
b. Using the largest field size will improve the spatial resolution.
c. Electronic magnification of the image (zoom) results in a lower patient dose.
d. The centre of the image is brighter than the periphery and this variation is called vignetting.
e. There is minimal distortion across the whole field in the final image on the monitor.

9.4 **The following are true of image intensifier tubes:**

a. There is a voltage of 25 kV between the photocathode and the anode.
b. The only source of brightness gain is by minification of the image.
c. Electrons from the photocathode are accelerated to the output screen via a series of dynodes.
d. The image intensifier shield is metal solely for added mechanical strength.
e. An aluminium layer prevents light from the output phosphor reactivating the input phosphor.

9.5 **When imaging with an image intensifier using automatic brightness control:**

a. Using a TV camera which demonstrates a low degree of lag reduces quantum noise in the image.
b. Selecting a higher dose rate or mA will reduce quantum noise in the image.
c. Using an x-ray field that extends beyond the edge of the patient may result in loss of image quality.
d. Pulsed fluoroscopy can reduce patient dose.
e. Pulsed fluoroscopy increases quantum noise in the image.

9.1 Answers

a. **True** – for a larger diameter image intensifier the output screen is often larger, 3.5 cm is more typical.

b. **True** – the electrons accelerated from the photocathode interact with the ZnCdS screen converting their kinetic energy into light photons.

c. **True** – this is an advantage of the needle-like shape of its crystals, which act as a light guide, preventing dispersion that would normally occur in a thick crystal.

d. **False** – the photocathode receives light photons from the input phosphor. It emits electrons – around 500 per x-ray photon absorbed in the input phosphor.

e. **False** – a fast film–screen system may have a spatial resolution exceeding 5 lpmm^{-1}. A typical image intensifier has a spatial resolution of 3–4 lpmm^{-1} but a TV monitor cannot present this level of detail and usually has a spatial resolution less than 2.5 lpmm^{-1}.

9.2 Answers

a. **False** – 10–20 mGy per minute.

b. **True** – 10–20 mGy per minute is 166–333 µGy per second. The input dose rates are usually between 0.1 and 1 µGy per second, so a factor of 300 is quite a conservative estimate.

c. **True** – the quantum sink is the point in the imaging system that determines the minimum number of information carriers that will contribute to the image. The lower the number of x-ray photons required the higher the level of quantum noise recorded in the final image (e.g. in a fast screen). If there is significant noise in this first step of information capture it cannot be corrected at a later stage by amplification.

d. **True**.

e. **False** – more than 100 000 light photons are produced for each absorbed x-ray photon.

9.3 Answers

a. **False** – the main limit on tube current is patient dose restriction.

b. **False** – using the smallest field magnifies the image, which improves spatial resolution.

c. **False** – because the x-ray beam is focused on a smaller area of the input phosphor minification is less effective at increasing brightness. Automatic controls adjust the crossover point of the electron beam in the intensifier to allow the whole of the output phosphor to be used. To counter the reduction in signal intensity to the output screen, x-ray intensity to the input phosphor must rise to maintain image brightness. This results in an increased patient dose.

d. True – this is caused by the effect of the inverse square law on reducing x-ray intensity at the periphery of the convex image intensifier input screen and by limitations of electron focusing by the electric field from the focusing elements in the image intensifier.

e. False – a test object (e.g. straight wire) will appear curved when placed at the edge of the input screen. The input screen is curved to attempt to limit this effect. Quality assurance tools to measure this include the Leeds Test Objects (developed by ARC and colleagues).

9.4 Answers

a. True – this acts to accelerate electrons emitted by the photocathode and intensifies the image produced when they collide with the output phosphor.

b. False – minification and electron acceleration increase brightness by about 100 fold each.

c. False – dynode chains are used in photomultiplier tubes. The amplification in an image intensifier requires the electrons to move along a direct path to preserve the spatial image.

d. False – the metal shield also acts as a radiation shield (it is usually lined with lead for this reason) and is earthed to prevent electric shock.

e. True – aluminium allows electrons from the photocathode to pass through it but stops light photons being emitted back towards the photocathode.

9.5 Answers

a. False – temporal averaging of the image results from the slow response of a camera sensor layer, one with a high amount of lag. This allows more photons to contribute to the image and reduces the effect of noise.

b. True – at the expense of increased patient dose.

c. True – part of the beam will be unattenuated by the patient, and this will result in areas of the image being very bright. Averaging of the brightness over the whole image may result in the relevant part of the image being too dark. This is one reason why proper collimation is important.

d. True – x-rays are switched on for only a fraction of the time. Despite the higher tube current used during each pulse, if the acquired frame rate is reduced, there may be a reduced patient dose.

e. False – the high dose rates used during each pulse means that there is no increase in noise. The penalty that is paid for the reduced patient dose is in the less frequent updating of the image, which can result in a jerky image of moving structures.

10. Computed tomography scanning

10.1 In computed tomography:

    a. Iterative reconstruction is commonly used in modern scanners.
    b. A window level of 20 is useful for bone imaging.
    c. The Hounsfield number of fat is about −100.
    d. A pixel in an image is a representation of the average linear attenuation coefficient of a voxel.
    e. The CT number of a voxel is determined only by the physical density of its contents.

10.2 In CT scanning:

    a. 5 mm copper filters are used.
    b. Only the detectors rotate in fourth generation machines.
    c. The spatial resolution is not limited by the pixel size and number.
    d. Image noise is increased by using a faster scan time (keeping all other exposure factors the same).
    e. Typical kVp setting is around 120 kV.

10.3 Regarding CT:

    a. It may be considered low dose equipment.
    b. It produces images with minimum detectable contrast of < 0.5%.
    c. Dose is linearly related to number of contiguous slices.
    d. The window width is the range of Hounsfield units covered by a structure.
    e. Use of narrow windows gives higher display contrast.

10.4 In CT:

    a. The spatial resolution is improved with a larger pixel size.
    b. Most interactions are due to Compton scatter.
    c. Images are produced with spatial resolution of 10 lpmm^{-1}.
    d. The quality of an image can be improved by increasing the pitch on a spiral CT.
    e. Thinner slices reduce the partial volume effect.

10.5 **Concerning modern CT scanners:**

a. They use several x-ray tubes to acquire data from different directions.
b. They use several hundred detector elements.
c. Each detector in a multislice scanner has its own collimator.
d. Pressurised xenon gas ionisation chambers are mainly used as detectors.
e. The detective quantum efficiency of a gas detector is better than that of a solid-state detector.

10.6 **In a CT image, noise:**

a. Can be measured as the standard deviation of the Hounsfield numbers for the image of a water phantom.
b. Is independent of mA, if all other factors are kept constant.
c. Is independent of scan time, if all other factors are kept constant.
d. Is inversely proportional to the square root of the dose.
e. Will make low contrast objects difficult to detect.

10.1 Answers

a. **False** – modified (filtered) back projection reconstruction is now used.

b. **False** – the useful range for imaging bone is 200–3000 Hounsfield units. The window level is the mean Hounsfield number displayed.

c. **True** – fat is represented by numbers in the range −50 to −200.

d. **True** – the voxel is the volume element in the patient addressed by the scanner.

e. **False** – the atomic number and the physical density both affect the attenuation.

10.2 Answers

a. **False** – 0.5 mm copper filters are typically used.

b. **False** – fourth generation scanners use a rotating x-ray tube and ring of stationary or fixed detectors.

c. **False** – the pixel size and number must match the resolving capacity of the rest of the system.

d. **True** – a shorter scan time would give less information, thereby increasing the amount of quantum noise, but with the benefit of reduced movement unsharpness.

e. **True**.

10.3 Answers

a. **False** – it is high dose equipment and is the main reason for the increasing contribution of radiation from medical examinations. However its use is justified by the superior information that is provided.

b. **True**.

c. **False** – the only dose-related quantity that will vary in this way is the dose–length product. Effective dose will vary with the number of slices, but as different slices may contain tissues with different weighting factors, the variation is not exactly linear. The absorbed dose at a point in the patient is dominated by the dose through the slice in which that point lies, and is almost independent of the number of slices. Indeed, CTDI is defined to be independent of the number of slices.

d. **False** – it is the range of Hounsfield units displayed in the image.

e. **True** – a narrow window must be used when a structure is only described by a small difference in the linear attenuation coefficient.

10.4 Answers

a. **False** – high contrast objects have better resolution if pixel size is decreased, within the limit of focal spot size, collimators, number and size of detectors, etc.

b. **True** – Compton scatter predominates over the kV range used in CT.

c. **False** – about 1 lp mm^{-1} for high contrast objects.

d. **False** – increasing the pitch increases the distance between interpolation points. This degrades spatial resolution in the longitudinal direction of movement and increases the probability of partial volume effects.

e. **True** – partial volume effect occurs because CT does not define detail within a voxel, but the average Hounsfield unit. If a high contrast object only partially occupies a volume, its attenuation coefficient will be averaged over the whole voxel, which results in a reduced Hounsfield unit in the pixel. This effect can be reduced by using thinner slices or smaller pixels to produce voxels that are less likely to be partially occupied.

10.5 Answers

a. **False** – one single x-ray tube.

b. **True** – or thousands depending on the scanner design.

c. **False**.

d. **False** –solid-state detectors are being used increasingly.

e. **False** – 60% vs. 80%.

10.6 Answers

a. **True** – or similar test phantom.

b. **False** – increasing mA means that more photons contribute to each pixel, reducing the relative variation of photons per pixel.

c. **False** – increasing scan time reduces noise by increasing the number of photons per pixel.

d. **True** – assuming that dose is proportional to the number of photons (N), the standard deviation will be the square root of N. The amount of noise is proportional to $\sqrt{N}/N$ (i.e. proportional to $1/\sqrt{N}$).

e. **True** – at low contrast, the difference between pixel values is comparable with their random variations.

11. Radionuclide imaging

11.1 In nuclear medicine:

a. The photoelectric effect predominates when photon energy is above 1 MeV.

b. A beta particle is emitted when molybdenum-99 decays to technetium-99m.

c. If a radionuclide used for nuclear medicine emits both beta and gamma radiation, the beta radiation will always give the greater dose.

d. Technetium-99m is a commonly used radionuclide because of its gamma ray energy emission of 300 keV.

e. The radiopharmaceutical ideally should have the shortest possible half-life.

11.2 In radioisotope imaging of body organs:

a. The effective half-life of the radionuclide depends more on its biological half-life than its radioactive half-life.

b. The spatial resolution is comparable to that of images produced by CT scanners.

c. The collimator contributes to the limitation of spatial resolution.

d. Little information can be gained regarding organ function.

e. The absorbed dose resulting from a radionuclide study is inversely proportional to its effective half-life.

11.3 A radionuclide for use in organ imaging should have:

a. A high photon energy (over 300 keV).

b. No alpha particulate emission.

c. High tumour to background ratio.

d. Multiple gamma peaks.

e. Low critical organ uptake.

11.4 Reasons for using technetium-99m (Tc-99m) in radionuclide imaging are:

a. It decays by beta(+) decay to Tc-99.

b. It has a short half-life and can be produced from a generator.

c. It is the cheapest radioisotope.

d. Its gamma ray energy emission minimises absorption within the body.

e. A Tc-99m generator can be used for up to 3 months before changing it.

11.5 Regarding technetium-99m:

a. The HVL in lead for 140 keV gamma rays is approximately 3 mm.
b. Its half-life is 10 hours.
c. The equivalent dose received by patient from a 600 MBq Tc-99m bone scan is about 4 mSv.
d. It is used for a variety of investigations including bone scans, renal studies and cerebral blood flow imaging.
e. It should be injected by an ARSAC licence holder.

11.6 Regarding photomultiplier tubes:

a. They may be used in contamination monitors with scintillation detectors.
b. They contain a photocathode which emits x-rays when light falls on it.
c. They require a potential difference of 30 volts across the tube.
d. The signal is amplified by a series of dynodes.
e. They contain an inert gas at a low pressure.

11.7 Regarding the gamma camera:

a. The primary function of the collimator is to remove scattered radiation.
b. A pulse height analyser can be used to detect two different nuclides simultaneously.
c. The crystal is made of caesium iodide (CsI), doped with thallium.
d. Spatial resolution and system sensitivity are directly related to each other.
e. An image with a total of 2000 measured counts is typical for a good definition image.

11.8 Flood field testing of a gamma camera:

a. Tests the spatial resolution of the system.
b. Is performed by imaging a large area source of Tc-99m or a similar radionuclide.
c. Typical system uniformity is 1%.
d. Uniformity is dependent on count rate.
e. A cracked crystal will not show as a defect.

11.9 **Regarding the dose received from radioactive material:**

a. The dose to the patient depends on the biological half-life.
b. The dose is inversely proportional to the radioactivity administered.
c. The dose to the patient is affected by the route of administration.
d. The dose is decreased the longer the image acquisition time.
e. The dose of a thallium myocardial scan is approximately 20 mSv.

11.10 **The dose used for a radionuclide study is designed to be:**

a. Less than published Diagnostic Reference Levels.
b. Approximately equal to the natural background radiation level.
c. Not more than 1 mSv.
d. Comparable to a CT scan of the same area.
e. The same as the occupational dose limit for classified workers.

11.11 **In radionuclide scanning the activity administered to the patient depends on:**

a. The weight of the subject.
b. The method of administration.
c. The half-life of the radionuclide used.
d. The gamma ray abundance of the radioactive isotope.
e. The metabolic pathway.

11.12 **Regarding radionuclide safety in nuclear medicine investigations:**

a. Generally, as the activity is low, no special precautions need be taken administering radionuclides to women of reproductive age.
b. A high activity patient should be treated on a general ward as an inpatient.
c. A high activity patient needing emergency surgery must be refused an operation, as the surgeon would be at increased risk of radiation exposure.
d. Solid waste from a high activity patient should be disposed of by incineration at the hospital.
e. All radionuclides must be administered in a controlled area.

11.1 Answers

a. **False** – the probability of photoelectric interactions is inversely proportional to the cube of the photon energy, so at such high energies its contribution will be negligible.

b. **True**.

c. **False** – this will depend on the relative abundance and energy of the beta and gamma radiation, so the gamma contribution might well be greater. Beta radiation is undesirable because it plays no part in image formation.

d. **False** – the gamma energy is 140 keV, and technetium has other properties that make it good for imaging.

e. **False** – the half-life should be suitable for the examination.

11.2 Answers

a. **False** – where one of the half-lives is much shorter than the other, the shorter one will predominate. If the half-lives are approximately equal, each will have an approximately equal effect.

b. **False** – the system has a resolution of about 1 lpcm^{-1}, CT spatial resolution for high contrast objects is about 1 lpmm^{-1}.

c. **True** – the intrinsic resolution is about 2–4 lpmm^{-1}, which is the resolution of the crystal alone. The system resolution includes that of the collimators, reducing resolution to around 1 lpcm^{-1}.

d. **False** – functional information is one of the major advantages of radionuclide imaging.

e. **False** – the dose will be greater for materials with a longer effective half-life.

11.3 Answers

a. **False** – between 100 and 300 keV ideally.

b. **True** – the dose from alpha radiation would be unacceptable. There are no alpha-emitting radionuclides that are used for imaging.

c. **True** – to provide an image with good contrast.

d. **False** – for detection of the primary gamma ray, a single gamma peak is preferred. All other photon energies detected can then be rejected as scatter.

e. **False** – the radionuclide should concentrate in the organ of interest, giving a high critical organ uptake.

11.4 Answers

a. False – it decays by isomeric transition from the excited state of Tc-99m to Tc-99, and emits a 140 keV gamma ray in the process.

b. True – its half-life is 6 hours, so it decays to a negligible activity within a relatively short time after the examination. It is produced in a generator from its parent Mo-99, which has a sufficiently long half-life to provide technetium for a week or so.

c. False – it is chosen for its properties not its cost.

d. True – 140 keV gamma rays are emitted.

e. False – it must be changed every week. Mo-99 has a half-life of 67 hours, so after a week its activity will be reduced by a factor of 6. After 3 months the activity would be reduced by a factor of over 10^9.

11.5 Answers

a. False – 0.3 mm.

b. False – 6 hours.

c. True.

d. True – labelled to different compounds it can be directed to different parts of the body.

e. False – the person administering the dose must be a trained operator, as defined in IRMER. The ARSAC licence holder is also the IRMER practitioner. The practitioner must justify the exposure but need not administer it.

11.6 Answers

a. True – they are also used in gamma cameras to amplify the light signal from the detector crystal.

b. False – the photocathode emits electrons.

c. False – a high potential difference of about 1200 volts is applied for acceleration of the electrons.

d. True – the dynodes are at increasing potential. At each one, the number of electrons is increased, producing a cascade effect.

e. False – the components are inside an evacuated glass envelope.

11.7 Answers

a. **False** – the primary function is to accept radiation travelling in the direction of the holes and allow the pulse arithmetic circuit to locate its origin. The collimator cannot differentiate between primary and scattered radiation.

b. **True** – if they emit different gamma energies.

c. **False** – it is made of sodium iodide, doped with thallium. CsI is used in image intensifiers.

d. **False** – they are inversely related. To improve resolution, the origin of each photon must be more precisely located. This is achieved by using a collimator with longer thinner holes, to restrict the photons accepted to those within a narrow angle of the aperture. Such a collimator rejects more photons, so that the resulting sensitivity is reduced. A thinner crystal improves resolution, because the photons emerging from the collimator cannot diverge as much. A thinner crystal is a less efficient detector, so sensitivity is again reduced.

e. **False** – approximately 500 000 is a typical count.

11.8 Answers

a. **False** – it tests the uniformity of the system, and should be carried out daily.

b. **True** – the source must be larger than the field of view. Specially constructed sources using cobalt-57 are normally used, though an alternative is a flat sealed box containing a solution of Tc-99m. It is measured with the source against the face of the camera, without and with the collimator in place, to test for both crystal and system non-uniformity respectively.

c. **True**.

d. **True** – at too low a count rate there will not be enough information for a uniform image.

e. **False** – it will appear as a linear defect.

11.9 Answers

a. **True** – the biological half-life determines how quickly the radioisotope is eliminated from the body and, together with the radioactive half-life, determines the effective half-life of the material.

b. **False** – the dose will be directly proportional to the activity.

c. **True** – injected material will not be taken up by tissues in the same way as orally administered or inhaled material. The effective dose, which depends on the doses to different tissues, is likely to be different.

d. **False** – the dose relates to the type and quantity of radioisotope administered, not to image acquisition time.

e. **True** – typically an effective dose of 18 mSv is quoted.

11.10 Answers

a. True – for nuclear medicine scans, the recommended maximum administered activities are those in the ARSAC guidance, found in the MARS Regulations. The values in the guidance have been adopted as diagnostic reference levels.

b. False – the background radiation level varies widely in different locations, and is useful only as an analogy for explaining doses, not as an indicator of a suitable dose for a study.

c. False – no dose limits exist for patients.

d. False – the dose for a different investigation might influence your choice of investigation, but an appropriate dose cannot be extrapolated from the dose received by using a different imaging modality.

e. False – there are no dose limits for investigations. The dose (or administered activity) for a study should be as low as practicable to achieve the required outcome. Therefore, of the options listed above, only the diagnostic reference level is relevant, since it is based on what is achievable in good practice.

11.11 Answers

a. True – the dose is increased in larger patients.

b. True – route of administration affects uptake of the radionuclide.

c. True – for a very short half-life material, a greater activity may need to be administered to ensure that sufficient is present throughout the scan. Using a very long half-life material (compared with Tc-99m) would not reduce the activity needed by much, since scans are done soon after injection. It would, though, greatly increase the dose to the patient.

d. True – the abundance is defined as the proportion of decays that result in the emission of a gamma ray.

e. True – this determines the biological half-life and determines the time that radioactivity is present in the body.

11.12 Answers

a. False – all females of childbearing age should be counselled and advised regarding pregnancy, breastfeeding and the timing of future conception.

b. False – high activity patients should have a single room, appropriate designation of areas, precautions for staff, carers etc. Patients having diagnostic investigations are normally 'low activity' and they can be treated on a general ward, or discharged.

c. False – the saving of life or alleviation of serious illness would justify the increased risk. The activity of the patient must be ascertained, and the radiation protection adviser (RPA) consulted about protection of the staff. Any surgery could be postponed if it is non-urgent.

d. False – the disposal route is determined by the hospital's waste disposal authorisation. Normally such waste is stored until activity has decayed to a low enough level to allow it to be transferred to an authorised contractor for disposal.

e. False – the need for a controlled area will be determined by the radiation and contamination levels that may exist. A controlled area may not be necessary.

12. Radiation protection

12.1 Biological effects of electromagnetic radiation are:

a. Different for an x-ray and a gamma ray of the same energy.
b. Attributed to the production of free radicals in tissue.
c. More severe in cells with a low turnover.
d. Enhanced by tissue hypoxia.
e. More severe if the radiation dose is fractionated.

12.2 Deterministic (non-stochastic) effects:

a. The $LD_{50/30}$ is the lethal dose required to kill 30% of a population at 50 days.
b. For a single exposure a whole body dose of 1 Gy is sufficient to cause haematopoietic syndrome.
c. The threshold is the same for all tissues.
d. The severity of the effect is directly proportional to the dose received.
e. The probability of occurrence is proportional to the dose received.

12.3 The following are examples of deterministic (non-stochastic) effects of radiation:

a. Erythema.
b. Myxoedema.
c. Basal cell carcinoma.
d. Sacro-iliitis.
e. Leukaemia.

12.4 Entrance surface dose:

a. May be expressed in gray.
b. May be expressed in rad.
c. Is absorbed dose.
d. Is decreased at high mAs.
e. May be measured using a thermoluminescent dosimeter.

12.5 **The following statements regarding radiation are true:**

a. The linear energy transfer (LET) is a measure of the heat energy absorbed by the tissues along the track of the radiation.
b. An average absorbed dose of 20 mGy from an x-ray beam would result in an equivalent dose of 20 mSv.
c. The radiation weighting factor for alpha particles is 20 times that of photons.
d. High energy neutrons have a radiation weighting factor of 5.
e. Radiation weighting factors are measured in sieverts.

12.6 **The gray:**

a. Is the unit of effective dose.
b. Can be used to measure skin dose.
c. Is preferred to the sievert when measuring dose from gamma radiation.
d. Is the unit used in the measurement of kerma.
e. Is equal to one joule per kilogram.

12.7 **The term exposure is:**

a. Defined in terms of the quantity of ionisation produced in air.
b. Applicable to all forms of ionising radiation.
c. Measured in sieverts.
d. Measured in terms of coulombs per kilogram.
e. The same as dose area product.

12.8 **An effective dose of 6 mSv:**

a. Is approximately 10 times the annual background radiation dose in the UK.
b. Received by a 17 year old trainee radiation worker in 1 year would require them to be classified.
c. Is a typical effective dose for a dental radiograph.
d. Carries a risk of fatal cancer of about 1 in 3000.
e. Is a typical effective dose for a barium meal examination.

12.9 **Regarding effective dose:**

a. The tissue weighting factor is measured in mSv.
b. For a given value of effective dose, the risk of a stochastic effect does not depend on which tissues are irradiated.
c. Skin and oesophagus have the same tissue weighting factor.
d. The tissue weighting factor for the breast is the same as that for the colon.
e. The tissue weighting factor for testes is 0.2.

12.10 **Concerning radiation protection:**

a. Medical exposures to patients are a minor factor in the total dose to the population at large from all sources.
b. The entrance surface dose to the body is the same as the effective dose.
c. Local rules are not a statutory requirement unless a dose limit may be exceeded.
d. The dose limit for the lens of the eye of a trainee aged 17 years is 150 mSv per year.
e. The risk of a stochastic effect to a radiation worker is greater than that of a deterministic effect.

12.11 **A radiation film badge:**

a. Does not contain an intensifying screen.
b. The sensitivity of dosimetry badges is uniform across a batch.
c. Can measure effective dose.
d. Contains an aluminium (dural) filter which stops beta particles.
e. Must be worn by anybody who may come into contact with ionising radiation.

12.12 **Film badges:**

a. Should be renewed every 6 months.
b. Cannot detect a radiation dose below 2 mGy.
c. If wearing a lead apron, the film badge should be worn over the lead apron.
d. Heating affects the latent image.
e. Are particularly useful when estimating extremity dose during interventional procedures.

12.13 **Thermoluminescent dose meters:**

a. Require the photon energy to be known in order to get a dose estimate.
b. Provide information about photon energy if a single TLD element is used.
c. Are more expensive than film badges.
d. Can be used to measure patient doses.
e. Are suitable for measuring breast doses in mammographic examinations.

12.14 In connection with the clinical use of ionising radiation:

   a. The dose to a single organ of a patient undergoing diagnostic imaging should not exceed 50 mSv in a year.
   b. Thermoluminescent dosimetry is only useful for monitoring staff.
   c. A PA chest x-ray results in a comparable dose to the patient as 1 month of average background radiation in the UK.
   d. A barium enema results in about the same dose to the patient as 3–4 years of average background radiation in the UK.
   e. Patient dose from a CT head scan is comparable to a year's annual background radiation dose in the UK.

12.15 Regarding entrance surface dose:

   a. In diagnostic x-ray exposures, the entrance surface dose is always numerically higher than the effective dose.
   b. A conventional lumbar spine x-ray has a higher entrance dose than a PA chest x-ray.
   c. Film badges are frequently used to estimate patient entrance surface dose rate.
   d. It is a good indicator of stochastic effects.
   e. It increases directly with the mAs.

12.16 Entrance dose:

   a. Is the absorbed dose at the surface of the patient's skin at the point where the x-ray enters the patient.
   b. It is unaffected by grid ratio.
   c. If the mAs is unchanged, it increases in proportion to the fourth power of the tube kV.
   d. It increases with the square root of the focus to skin distance.
   e. With higher kV and the same degree of film blackening, the skin dose is increased.

12.17 Regarding dose area product:

   a. It is independent of the distance from the source.
   b. It is measured in mGy.
   c. It can be used to estimate effective dose to the patient.
   d. It is measured using an ionisation chamber, which completely intercepts the x-ray beam.
   e. Dose area product meters are mandatory on all x-ray equipment.

12.18 Regarding radiation protection of staff:

a. If required during fluoroscopy a thyroid shield of 3.5 mm lead equivalent should be worn by the operator.
b. Wall radiation shielding in a general x-ray room should be around 2 mm lead equivalent.
c. A 0.25 mm lead apron will transmit approximately 0.2% of x-rays generated by a tube at 50 kV.
d. In fluoroscopy, staff dose rates tend to be lower when using an undercouch tube compared to an overcouch tube.
e. The clear protective screen within x-ray rooms should be about 20 mm lead glass equivalent.

12.19 A spill, onto the floor, of 0.1% of a typical bone scan activity of technetium-99m (500 MBq):

a. Would easily be detected by a Geiger counter.
b. Would produce an insignificant level of surface contamination if spread over an area of 1000 cm^2.
c. Should be reported to the regulatory authorities.
d. Will not be detectable after 24 hours.
e. Would be unlikely to produce measurable readings on the personnel dose meters of staff.

12.1 Answers

a. **False** – they have the same linear energy transfer, which is the density of ionisation along the path of the radiation. X-rays and gamma rays are not distinguishable in terms of their properties.

b. **True** – this indirect damage is produced by the ionisation of water molecules and is more common than direct damage by the radiation to covalent bonds. The free radical produces chemical modifications in solute organic molecules, which starts a chain reaction of events, leading to biological damage.

c. **False** – tissues with a high cell turnover (replication rate) are more likely to be damaged (e.g. gastrointestinal tract and haematopoietic stem cells). This was first described by Bergonié and Tribondeau in 1906.

d. **False** – a high oxygen tension enhances low linear energy transfer effects (e.g. beta and gamma irradiation).

e. **False** – for deterministic effects, repair and recovery can occur if given sufficient time between irradiations. This principle is used when administering higher doses of radiation over a fractionated course in radiotherapy.

12.2 Answers

a. **False** – this is the amount needed to kill 50% of the population at 30 days.

b. **True** – this is the approximate threshold dose for symptoms. Subclinical effects will occur at lower doses. The LD_{50} is about 2.5–5 Gy.

c. **False** – temporary impairment of fertility may be seen at doses as low as 150 mGy, whereas gastrointestinal syndrome is not seen until 3–4 Gy is received. Effects on the central nervous system require even greater doses.

d. **False** – although severity increases with dose, it is not directly proportional to it.

e. **False** – although this is thought to be the case for stochastic effects.

12.3 Answers

a. **True** – early transient erythema is seen after 2–3 Gy, and radiation burns are seen after about 10 Gy.

b. **True**.

c. **False** – a stochastic effect.

d. **False** – historically people with ankylosing spondylitis were treated using radiotherapy.

e. **False** – a stochastic effect.

12.4 Answers

a. True – entrance surface dose is the absorbed dose measured at the skin surface, so the gray is an appropriate unit.

b. True – the rad is the old, non-SI unit of absorbed dose. It is still sometimes used in the USA. (1 Gy = 100 rad).

c. True – entrance surface dose is absorbed dose measured in air at the surface of a patient.

d. False – increasing the mAs increases the total number of x-ray photons in the beam, which increases the entrance surface dose.

e. True.

12.5 Answers

a. False – the LET is a measure of the rate of energy transfer (all processes) to the medium per track length. The prime method of transfer is by ionisation processes rather than by direct heating. Radiation with a low linear energy transfer would pass through the tissue easily, whereas radiation with a higher linear energy transfer would be absorbed.

b. True – the equivalent dose is the average absorbed dose in a tissue multiplied by a weighting factor for the type of radiation. Where there is more than one type of radiation, the equivalent doses from each are summed.

c. True – see d.

d. False – the radiation weighting factor varies with the type and energy of the radiation. High energy neutrons and alpha particles have a weighting factor of 20. Low energy neutrons are 5. Beta particles, gamma and x-ray photons have a weighting factor of 1.

e. False – they have no unit.

12.6 Answers

a. False – the sievert is the unit of effective dose.

b. True – it is a unit of absorbed dose.

c. False – the sievert and the gray are both appropriate units for measuring dose. The absorbed dose (measured in gray) and the equivalent dose (sievert) for a gamma beam are identical as gamma rays have a radiation weighting factor of 1.

d. True – kerma is kinetic energy released per unit mass. It is measured in Jkg^{-1}, which is the same as gray.

e. True.

12.7 Answers

a. **True** – it is the sum of all of the charges of one sign produced in air when all the electrons produced in a unit mass have been completely stopped in air.

b. **False** – it is defined only for photons.

c. **False** – the SI unit is the coulomb per kilogram, though the older unit roentgen may still be used ($1\ R = 2.58 \times 10^{-4} Ckg^{-1}$).

d. **True**.

e. **False**.

12.8 Answers

a. **False** – annual background radiation is approximately 2.2 mSv in the UK.

b. **False** – according to the regulations (IRR99), trainees may not be classified. 6 mSv is the dose limit for trainees, so although the limit has not quite been exceeded, the dose should trigger an investigation and a change in working practices. An employee expected to receive 6 mSv in a year must be classified.

c. **False** – it is usually less than 0.01 mSv.

d. **True** – risk of a fatal cancer is about 5% per Sv, making the risk from 6 mSv about 1 in 3000.

e. **False** – less than half of this would be a typical dose, although 6 mSv is within the range of doses encountered.

12.9 Answers

a. **False** – it has no units.

b. **True** – the effective dose takes tissue sensitivity into account by means of the weighting factors. So, ignoring the uncertainties inherent in the weighting factors, the estimated risk is independent of the tissues irradiated.

c. **False** – see e.

d. **False** – see e.

e. **True** – for lung, stomach, colon and bone marrow it is 0.12, the oesophagus, thyroid, breast, bladder and liver have a weighting factor of 0.05 and skin is grouped with cortical bone and has a value of 0.01.

12.10 Answers

a. **False** – medical radiation contributes approximately 14% of total background radiation in the UK.
b. **False** – the effective dose is calculated from the absorbed doses to the different tissues, multiplied by their weighting factors. The entrance dose is a measure of the absorbed dose at the surface of the patient.
c. **False** – local rules are required if there are controlled areas, as laid out in IRR 1999.
d. **False** – the dose limits are 50 mSv per annum for a trainee aged 16–18 years and 150 mSv per annum for an adult classified worker.
e. **True** – if the dose limits are adhered to deterministic effects are avoided.

12.11 Answers

a. **True** – double emulsion film is used without a screen.
b. **True** – provided they are correctly stored and developed.
c. **False** – the badge gives information on the type of radiation and the absorbed dose at the position that the badge was worn. However, it cannot give information on the distribution of dose throughout the body, so it cannot measure effective dose. Effective dose may be inferred from film badge readings by assuming the reading represents a uniform whole-body dose.
d. **True** – though the function of the dural filter is not simply to stop beta particles. In conjunction with the other filters it also enables the photon energy to be estimated.
e. **False** – the need for personal monitoring depends on the type of work being done and will be determined by a risk assessment. Even for a classified worker, a film badge might not be the most appropriate way of assessing dose. Dose assessment is a legal requirement for a classified person.

12.12 Answers

a. **False** – every month or as written in the local rules. It is impracticable to issue them for periods greater than 2 months. If left for too long a time the latent image may fade.
b. **False** – the minimum detectable dose level is about 0.2 mGy.
c. **False** – otherwise the film-badge dose will overestimate the actual dose received.
d. **True** – increased humidity/temperature leads to fog formation affecting the latent image. This could be misinterpreted as a higher radiation dose.
e. **False** – thermoluminescent dosimeters come in many different shapes and sizes, and can be applied to fingertips and forehead (for retinal dose). Film badges cannot be used for this.

12.13 Answers

a. **False** – the variation in response with energy is small enough to allow a dose estimate to be made without knowing the energy.

b. **False** – a single TLD can provide only a single reading of dose. To obtain information on energy a monitoring badge would have to contain several TLD elements, each under a different filter.

c. **True** – but they can be used repeatedly. This makes the costs of commercial services similar, whether using film or TLD.

d. **True** – they can be attached to the patient in the x-ray beam.

e. **False** – at the low photon energies used in mammography they would be visible on the image.

12.14 Answers

a. **False** – no dose limits exist for patients.

b. **False** – it is used in staff and where necessary patient monitoring.

c. **False** – the annual background radiation dose in the UK is around 2.4 mSv, so a dose of 0.02 mSv, typical for a chest x-ray, is equivalent to around 3 days' background radiation.

d. **True** – resulting in an effective dose of about 7 mSv.

e. **True** – a CT head scan results in an effective dose of about 2–2.5 mSv.

12.15 Answers

a. **True** – e.g. a typical PA chest x-ray entrance dose is 0.2 mGy, and the effective dose 0.02 mSv. Effective dose is calculated from the absorbed doses to the various tissues in the body. Some of these will lie outside the radiation beam and receive very little dose. Even those in the main beam will receive a dose smaller than the entrance dose because of attenuation.

b. **True** – typical values for a chest x-ray are 0.2 mGy compared with 4–10 mGy for a lumbar spine.

c. **False** – thermoluminescent dose meters are used when necessary for this.

d. **False** – skin dose alone does not allow calculation of the effective dose. However, it is a good predictor of deterministic (non-stochastic) effects.

e. **True** – as x-ray output increases directly with mAs.

12.16 Answers

a. **True** – it is usually defined as the absorbed dose (including backscatter) measured in air at the surface of the patient.

b. **False** – increased grid ratio necessitates higher exposure.

c. **False** – it is approximately proportional to the square of the tube kV.

d. **False** – it decreases with the square of the focus to skin distance.

e. **False** – the beam is more penetrating, so a smaller skin dose will achieve the same film dose.

12.17 Answers

a. **True** – it is constant at any distance from the source. As the x-ray beam gets further away from the source, it diverges. The area covered by the beam increases, but the dose decreases, as there are fewer x-rays per unit area.

b. **False** – it is dose $\times$ area and is measured in $mGy\,cm^2$, or $Gy\,cm^2$.

c. **True** – either by estimating the energy imparted to the patient, or by using tables published by the National Radiological Protection Board to approximate the effective dose.

d. **True** – the reading from the ionisation chamber has to reflect the beam size. It can only do this if the beam always lies entirely within the chamber.

e. **False** – however, IRMER requires new equipment to give an indication of the radiation delivered. In some cases a post-exposure reading of the kV and mAs is sufficient to comply.

12.18 Answers

a. **False** – the need for a thyroid shield will be determined by a risk assessment, but if required a 0.25–0.5 mm thick shield is adequate.

b. **True** – a similar degree of protection from scattered radiation could be achieved from 15 mm barium plaster or 150 mm concrete.

c. **True**.

d. **True** – they are highest with an overcouch tube for three reasons. First, the entrance plane is at the top of the patient, so backscatter is in the direction of the upper body of nearby staff rather than toward the lower limbs – an important consideration in fluoroscopy. Second, any palpation of the patient (not recommended for overcouch tubes) would be on the entrance side, where the dose is greatest. Finally, it is simpler to shield around the intensifier with an undercouch tube, than to shield around the tube when the tube is overcouch.

e. **False** – about 2 mm thick is sufficient.

12.19 Answers

a. **True** – the activity spilt would be about 0.5 MBq. Even with a detection efficiency of 1%, the instrument would probably detect about 1000 counts per second.

b. **False** – the contamination level would be about 500 Bq/cm^2. It is usual to aim for a contamination level of less than 30 Bq/cm^2 in public areas and 300 Bq/cm^2 in controlled areas.

c. **False** – it does not have to be reported.

d. **False** – 24 hours is 4 half-lives for technetium, leaving a detectable activity of about 30 kBq.

e. **True** – despite the high readings on contamination monitors, the dose rate at waist height would be only about 0.01 μSv/h. Therefore the total dose would be less than 0.1 μSv even if a person remained near the spill until the technetium had decayed completely.

13. Patient dosimetry

13.1 The dose, as measured at a point within the x-ray beam inside the patient, will be decreased by (assume the film density is kept constant):

a. Decreasing focal spot size.
b. Lowering kV.
c. Use of an anti-scatter grid.
d. Use of a fast screen.
e. Decreasing field size.

13.2 A device chosen to monitor the radiation received by a patient from an x-ray examination:

a. Should have a response that varies linearly with photon energy.
b. Must be as sensitive to x-rays as possible.
c. Must give a dose reading that is independent of field size.
d. Should not be visible on the x-ray image.
e. Must be the cheapest method available.

13.3 Ionisation chambers:

a. Can be used to measure exposure.
b. Are suitable for detection of individual particles and gamma rays.
c. Are suitable for radiation dosimetry because the response closely follows absorbed dose in tissue.
d. Do not require a highly stabilised voltage supply.
e. Give an output current very closely proportional to radiation intensity.

13.4 Properties of thermoluminescent (TL) monitors for dosimetry, compared with film, include:

a. Their response is not linear over a wide range of dose.
b. Their response (signal per unit dose) varies widely with energy.
c. The chip is heated to 2200°C during reading.
d. Annealing is required after readout.
e. They can measure doses from approximately 0.1 mGy to 10^4 Gy.

13.5 Regarding scintillation detectors:

a. The higher the incident photon energy the larger the resulting electronic pulse.
b. They cannot discriminate between different isotopes.
c. The detector size is inversely proportional to the sensitivity.
d. A thick detector is preferred for measuring beta radiation.
e. Detectors are inorganic crystals.

13.6 The Geiger–Müller tube:

a. Measures absorbed dose directly.
b. Is not used in dose rate monitors.
c. Contains a central thin wire cathode.
d. Requires a quenching agent.
e. Has a dead time of approximately 300 seconds.

13.7 The following are commonly used for the measurement of the radiation dose to patients from x-ray examinations:

a. A thermoluminescent dosimeter.
b. An ionisation chamber.
c. A scintillation counter.
d. A spinning top.
e. An aluminium step wedge.

13.1 Answers

a. **False** – focal spot size is unrelated to dose.

b. **False** – the film dose, and therefore the patient exit surface dose, must remain the same. Since attenuation of a lower kV beam will be greater, the dose at any point before the exit surface has to be greater.

c. **False** – the use of a grid increases dose, as some radiation is absorbed by the grid. The grid ratio should be as low as possible to minimise patient dose.

d. **True** – the higher the speed of the screen, the smaller the dose required to achieve the same film density. The fastest film–screen combination should be used consistent with an acceptable level of image quality.

e. **True** – with a smaller field size, a greater proportion (though not a greater number) of photons are scattered outside the volume of the main beam, reducing the dose slightly. This effect is not nearly as important for patient protection as the reduction in the volume of tissue irradiated. The field size is reduced by collimating the beam carefully, and should be smaller than the detector size to confirm collimation.

13.2 Answers

a. **False** – the response should be independent of energy.

b. **False** – it should have sufficient sensitivity to give a reading over the range of doses likely to be encountered.

c. **False** – although some devices work in this way, dose area product meters give a reading that is proportional to the area of the beam.

d. **True** – if the device appears in the image it might obscure parts of it, or appear as a lesion.

e. **False** – the most appropriate method should be used which should not be determined by cost.

13.3 Answers

a. **True** – exposure is defined in terms of charge per unit mass of air ($C\,kg^{-1}$). An air-filled or air equivalent ionisation chamber can measure the charge collected (current multiplied by time), and can therefore be calibrated in terms of exposure.

b. **False** – they produce a small current from the collection of all the ion pairs produced by the radiation. The contribution from an individual particle is too small to measure, and cannot be distinguished from the rest of the signal.

c. **True** – as the mean atomic number of air ($Z = 7.6$) is very close to that of muscle/soft tissue ($Z = 7.4$), the number of ionisation events in air is similar to that occuring in the same mass of tissue.

d. **True** – provided the voltage is great enough to prevent recombination of ions, and not great enough to cause amplification by accelerating electrons to cause further ionisations, the output is largely independent of voltage.

e. **True** – the number of ion pairs produced is proportional to the energy absorbed. Since absorbed dose is energy per unit mass, the current is proportional to absorbed dose.

13.4 Answers

a. **False** – they do demonstrate a linear response, unlike film. At very high doses an enhanced response causes a departure from the linear response, but this occurs outside the normal range of dose for which TL dosimetry is used.

b. **False** – there is some variation with energy (up to about 40%, depending on the type of TL material). The variation is small in comparison with that of film, which requires a holder containing filters to enable the dose to be measured.

c. **False** – reading is done at 200 to 300°C, causing the electrons to fall out of energy traps back to the ground state. Even when they are annealed, the temperature is only about 400°C.

d. **True** – to remove any stored images ready for reuse.

e. **True**.

13.5 Answers

a. **True** – the size of the electronic pulse depends on the energy absorbed when a photon interacts within the detector.

b. **False** – if a detector is used with pulse height measurement electronics, the photon energy can be measured, and this can be used to determine the isotope. Not all scintillator materials can be used in this way, and even those that can are often used as simple detectors.

c. **False** – the sensitivity increases with detector size. The number of interactions increases with the volume of material.

d. **False** – in scintillator materials, beta particles would be absorbed in the first few millimetres, so a thicker detector would not detect more radiation. Very thin detectors can be used to produce contamination monitors sensitive to beta particles, while being inefficient at stopping gamma rays. This allows them to measure beta radiation contamination in areas with high background gamma radiation.

e. **False** – a number of organic scintillators are available, including liquids used in the assay of very low energy beta emitting nuclides such as tritium.

13.6 Answers

a. **False** – it detects individual ionisation events as electronic pulses, which can be counted, but the pulse size is independent of energy. Absorbed dose is defined as energy absorbed per unit mass, which is not what is being measured in this case.

b. **False** – although they cannot be said to measure dose, G-M tubes are used in many dose-measuring instruments. They are often enclosed in a metal shield to provide some compensation for the variation of response with photon energy. They are then calibrated so that the reading is displayed in units of dose, and are a cheaper alternative to ionisation chambers.

c. **False** – the central wire is the anode.

d. **True** – alcohol or bromine is added to the counting gas (argon/helium) to prevent the discharge continuing before another pulse is detected.

e. **False** – the dead time is typically 300 microseconds and is the time taken following initiation of discharge for the voltage to recover sufficiently to allow another pulse to be produced. During this time no more detections can be made.

13.7 Answers

a. **True**.

b. **True** – a dose area product meter is an ionisation chamber.

c. **False** – although you can, in principle, measure dose with a scintillation counter, it is not practicable for patient doses.

d. **False** – this is used to check x-ray exposure times.

e. **False** – this is used to produce a range of densities on a film for quality assurance purposes.

14. UK Legislation – Statutory Requirements and Non-statutory Recommendations

14.1 **The Ionising Radiation Regulations 1999 (IRR 1999):**

a. Are a good practice guide and have no legal status in hospitals.
b. Apply primarily to patients.
c. Specify the dose limits.
d. State that the radiation protection adviser (RPA) is responsible for management of the safety of radiation workers.
e. State that regular quality assurance checks on medical radiation equipment are a legal requirement.

14.2 **The Medical and Dental Guidance notes issued to provide guidance on IRR 1999 include the following recommendations:**

a. For fixed equipment the film–focus distance cannot be less than 45 cm.
b. Body aprons should be worn with a protective equivalent of not less than 0.25 mm lead for use with x-rays up to 100 kVp.
c. The lead aprons and thyroid shields provide adequate protection from the primary beam.
d. There is a maximum recommended skin entrance dose rate for fluoroscopy of a standard patient.
e. A 0.25 mm lead filter should be used for normal diagnostic work.

14.3 **The Ionising Radiation Regulations 1999 (IRR 1999):**

a. State that classified workers should be subject to continuous dose assessment.
b. Define the terms 'controlled' and 'supervised' areas.
c. Are not applicable to radiation exposures involving radionuclides.
d. State that a supervised area is needed if any person is likely to receive 0.1 mSv per annum.
e. State that the radiation protection supervisor (RPS) should have physics training and be certified competent by the HSE.

14.4   Regarding controlled areas:

a. Only a classified person may enter a controlled area.
b. The entrance must have a warning sign and an indication of the nature of the hazard.
c. Controlled areas should be described in the local rules.
d. A controlled area may contain a window.
e. Radionuclides must be administered in a controlled area.

14.5   Concerning dose limits for employees over 18 years of age:

a. They are not applicable to classified workers.
b. A dose limit of 50 mSv in a single year may be acceptable providing the dose received over 5 years does not exceed 100 mSv.
c. The dose to the hand must not exceed 50 mSv per annum.
d. A dose of 20 mSv in a calendar year received by a person at their place of work must be investigated.
e. A confirmed single overexposure of 30 mSv must be investigated, and the report kept for 50 years.

14.6   Regarding dose limits:

a. Dose to the hands should be less than 10 times the whole body dose limit.
b. The annual dose limit to the skin is 500 mSv.
c. There is a limit of 10 mSv per annum for comforters and carers.
d. There is a limit of 10 mSv for the abdomen of a classified female worker of reproductive capacity in any consecutive 3 month interval.
e. They are independent of the type of radiation to which the person is exposed.

14.7   Regarding overexposure of patients:

a. Exposures much greater than intended resulting from equipment faults must be reported directly to the Health and Safety Executive.
b. An incident in which a patient receives 3 times the intended dose for a chest x-ray must be reported.
c. An incident in which a patient receives 5 times the intended dose for a CT abdomen should be reported.
d. An incident in which a patient receives 10 times the intended dose for a mammogram must be reported.
e. An incident in which a patient receives 1.5 times the intended dose for a treatment fraction in radiotherapy should be reported.

14.8   Concerning the Ionising Radiation (Medical Exposure) Regulations 2000:

a. They replace the Ionising Radiation (Protection of Persons Undergoing Medical Examination or Treatment) Regulations 1988.
b. The referring clinician must have adequate radiation training.
c. A nurse practitioner may not act as a referrer.
d. Radiopharmacists may act as operators.
e. The operator has the responsibility of ensuring that the procedure for ascertaining the possibility of pregnancy has been followed in a female patient of reproductive age, before carrying out an exposure.

14.9   The Ionising Radiation (Medical Exposure) Regulations 2000:

a. Are to help ensure staff receive a low occupational dose.
b. Require doctors who request x-rays to justify the examination.
c. State that the outcome of every exposure must be recorded.
d. Describe the training that operators must have.
e. State that the same person may not act as referrer, operator and practitioner.

14.10 Regarding diagnostic reference levels (DRL):

a. A patient DRL may be exceeded.
b. A DRL should always be expressed as dose area product.
c. A local DRL should be set higher than those nationally recommended.
d. The nationally proposed DRL for a PA chest x-ray is 0.3 mGy (entrance dose).
e. The European recommended DRL for a CT head scan is 60 mGy (CT dose index).

14.11 Radiation exposure of people for research benefit:

a. Should be subject to dose constraints.
b. The risks associated with the radiation exposure involved must be communicated to the volunteers.
c. If using radionuclides, an ARSAC certificate must be obtained for that procedure.
d. All medical research should be approved by the local research and ethics committee.
e. The number of volunteers involved may exceed that needed for statistical significance.

14.12 Regarding the Radioactive Substances Act 1993:

a. It controls the storage, use and disposal of radioactive substances.
b. It is enforced by the Health and Safety Executive.
c. Hospitals may keep any amount of radioactive substances without registration, under the Hospitals' Exemption Order.
d. A registration document, granted under the Act, imposes security conditions for storage of radioactive substances.
e. Administration of radioactive material to a patient is considered to be disposal of radioactivity.

14.13 Considering the Medicines (Administration of Radioactive Substances) Regulations (MARS) 1978:

a. ARSAC is an abbreviation for 'Advisors for Radioactive Substances and Cross-Sectional Imaging'.
b. To obtain an ARSAC licence the applicant needs to demonstrate adequate scientific support is available.
c. An ARSAC licence should be obtained by radiology registrars working in nuclear medicine.
d. The ARSAC clinical licences are valid for 5 years.
e. The licence covers all work involving radionuclides in all hospitals within a trust.

Answers

a. **False** – they are legally binding regulations.
b. **False** – they are mainly concerned with the protection of all people at a place of work, so patients who are not in the process of being x-rayed are regarded as 'any other person'. They do apply to patients undergoing medical exposures, but only in the event of equipment faults causing overexposures.
c. **True** – the limits apply to anybody at a place of work. It should be noted that the dose limit is not regarded as a safe dose, but one within which the risks of stochastic effects are deemed acceptable and deterministic effects are avoided.
d. **False** – the employer has overall responsibility for safety of workers. However almost all employers using ionising radiation will need to consult and appoint a suitable RPA, with relevant certification, knowledge and experience.
e. **True** – at suitable intervals.

14.2 Answers

a. **True** – ideally the FFD should be as large as possible to decrease patient dose. For fixed equipment the FFD should be at least 45 cm. For radiography of the chest, the distance should not be less than 60 cm. Smaller FFDs (30 cm and 45 cm) are permitted for mobile equipment.
b. **True** – 0.25 mm for up to 100 kVp, 0.35 mm for 100 kVp and over.
c. **False** – they only provide protection from scatter and the primary beam after it has passed through the patient.
d. **True** – this should not exceed 100 mGy per minute for all field sizes.
e. **False** – 2.5 mm aluminium equivalent is recommended.

14.3 Answers

a. **True** – and unclassified persons may also require dose assessment so the employer can show that their doses are low.
b. **True** – radiation areas are designated as controlled to ensure that exposures from radiation sources are properly restricted. Controlled areas must be established where people are likely to exceed 6 mSv per year, or where special procedures are needed to avoid this. A supervised area is one where any person is likely to receive over 1 mSv per year, or one tenth of any dose limit.
c. **False** – the regulations apply to all forms of ionising radiation.
d. **False** – 1 mSv or 10% of any equivalent dose limit in a year.
e. **False** – the RPS should be a senior person within a department (e.g. a superintendent radiographer) to help ensure compliance with the IRR 1999. The RPS should have some radiation protection training. HSE certification is not required.

14.4 Answers

a. **False** – other persons may enter in accordance with written arrangements (staff in hospitals are not usually classified). The regulations do not prevent patients from entering a controlled area to be x-rayed.

b. **True** – this should be at eye level and indicate, for example, the presence of x-radiation or unsealed sources. The sign may incorporate an indication of the personal protective equipment needed to enter.

c. **True**.

d. **True** – provided that the window does not result in conditions requiring a controlled area in a place that is not under the control of the employer, e.g. a visitors' coffee bar.

e. **False** – the status of the room where administration takes place depends on the amount of radioactivity to be handled and the outcome of a risk assessment.

14.5 Answers

a. **False** – the dose limits apply to all employees.

b. **True** – but the employer must notify the HSE if he/she intends to operate in this way, and demonstrate that he is 'restricting exposures so far as is reasonably practicable'.

c. **False** – extremity dose limit 500 mSv per annum.

d. **True** – the employer must carry out a formal investigation if a member of staff exceeds 15 mSv in a year. It is recommended that a lower local level is set to trigger an investigation. The report of the investigation must be kept for at least 2 years.

e. **True** – any confirmed overexposure exceeding a dose limit must be investigated, and the report kept for 50 years or until the person is aged 75.

14.6 Answers

a. **False** – the limits work out to 25 times the limit on effective dose for employees (the whole body dose limit is 20 mSv and the extremity dose limit 500 mSv) and for trainees (6 mSv and 150 mSv). It is 15 times this for other persons (1 mSv and 15 mSv). Extremity limits are not written as multiples of effective doses.

b. **True** – the limit applies to any 1 cm^2 of skin.

c. **False** – no dose limits exist for individuals who knowingly and willingly incur exposures to ionising radiation through the support of another person. However the National Radiological Protection Board (NRPB) recommended a constraint of 5 mSv for such episodes.

d. **False** – she must not receive more than 13 mSv in any 3 month period. However after the employer is notified of a pregnancy, conditions of exposure must be such that the dose to the fetus is unlikely to exceed 1 mSv.

e. **True** – the doses are effective/equivalent doses so the radiation type has already been accounted for.

14.7 Answers

a. **True** – equipment faults should also be reported to the Medical Devices Agency so that hazard warnings can be issued.
b. **False** – for low dose examinations, a report need not be made unless the dose exceeds that intended by a factor of 20. A report may be made at a lower dose, particularly if the incident could have resulted in a much greater exposure.
c. **True** – guidance defines 'much greater than intended' as more than 3 times the intended doses for high dose examinations.
d. **True** – a mammogram is, according to current guidance, a 'medium dose examination', where much greater than intended means an overexposure by a factor of 10.
e. **True** – overdoses for single fractions should be reported if they exceed the intended dose by more than 20%.

14.8 Answers

a. **True**.
b. **False** – the referrer does not need any radiation training.
c. **False** – IRMER defines a referrer as '… a registered medical or dental practitioner or other health professional who is entitled by the employer's procedures to refer individuals for medical exposure to a practitioner'. This definition may include trained nurse practitioners, physiotherapists, podiatrists, etc.
d. **True** – the operator is any person who carries out any practical part of a medical exposure. The person dispensing radionuclide injections is carrying out a 'practical aspect'.
e. **True** – by using the pregnancy enquiry procedure written in the employer's local rules.

14.9 Answers

a. **False** – the regulations contain no requirements relating to staff doses. Their aim is to ensure that doses to patients are appropriate, e.g. by the introduction of diagnostic reference levels and dose constraints.
b. **False** – the practitioner justifies the examination. The referrer is obliged to provide enough clinical information for the practitioner to justify the examination. Practitioners are usually clinical radiologists.
c. **True** – this may include the recording of factors relevant to patient dose.
d. **True** – and also that for practitioners.
e. **False** – e.g. a dentist is likely to fulfil all of these roles in an examination.

14.10 Answers

a. **True** – they are a guide to good practice for the 'standard' patient. For example, when imaging an obese patient, it may be necessary to exceed the DRL.

b. **False** – the most convenient and relevant measurement should be used, e.g. entrance dose, mAs, etc.

c. **False** – local levels may be lower than the recommended ones, but should not be higher.

d. **True** – at the time of writing.

e. **True** – but a locally set DRL may be different.

14.11 Answers

a. **True** – these must not be exceeded.

b. **True**.

c. **True** – these are normally valid for 2 years, or for the duration of the research project if this is shorter.

d. **True** – whether it involves ionising radiation or not.

e. **False**.

14.12 Answers

a. **True**.

b. **False** – the Environment Agency.

c. **False** – the exemption applies to the use of small quantities of radioactive materials in a hospital. A nuclear medicine department will usually use quantities in excess of the exemption limits, so the hospital will need to register under the Radioactive Substances Act.

d. **True**.

e. **True** – strictly speaking, it is the excretion of the activity that is the disposal.

14.13 Answers

a. **False** – Administration of Radioactive Substances Advisory Committee.

b. **True** – e.g., by showing that the procedures will be performed in a properly staffed and equipped nuclear medicine department.

c. **False** – generally, only consultant radiologists with experience in nuclear medicine are considered to have sufficient experience to hold a licence. They will usually act as the practitioner for all the nuclear medicine tests in that department.

d. **True** – research certificates are only valid for 2 years.

e. **False** – each licence is specific for named tests and an individual practitioner at a particular hospital.

Mock examination

Mark each question T (true) or F (false). Correct answers score 1 mark, incorrect answers score minus 1 mark, questions not attempted score 0.

Time allowed 75 minutes.

1. Concerning atomic structure:

    a. K shell electrons are bound more tightly to the nucleus than L shell electrons.
    b. Electron shells are associated with discrete energy levels.
    c. An element can have atoms with a range of atomic numbers.
    d. The diameter of an atom is about 10 times the diameter of the nucleus.
    e. There must be more neutrons than protons in the nucleus.

2. Regarding radioactivity:

    a. In beta (–) decay, the atomic number of the nucleus is increased.
    b. Positron (beta +) decay occurs in nuclei that have a deficit of neutrons compared with stable nuclei of the same element.
    c. Technetium-99m decays to molybdenum-99.
    d. Gamma rays are emitted with discrete energies.
    e. Beta particles are emitted with discrete energies.

3. With regard to Compton scatter:

    a. The initial photon energy is much greater than the electron binding energy.
    b. The energy lost by the photon depends only on the angle through which it is scattered.
    c. The electron may be scattered through angles up to 180°.
    d. Compton scatter has no effect on image contrast.
    e. It becomes more probable as photon energy increases.

4. **If an x-ray tube is operated with a high frequency generator, then compared with the same tube operated with a full wave, single phase generator:**

   a. The maximum energy of the x-rays will be increased.
   b. The x-ray output will be increased.
   c. The half value thickness of the x-ray beam will be increased.
   d. The mean energy of the x-rays will be increased.
   e. The anode heel effect will be more pronounced.

5. **In a mammographic x-ray tube:**

   a. There may be more than one target.
   b. The tube voltage is typically 35–45 kV.
   c. The axial ray is directed to the centre of the x-ray field.
   d. The anode does not rotate.
   e. The focal spot size is typically 0.6 mm.

6. **Concerning anti-scatter grids:**

   a. With a parallel grid, cut off limits the maximum field size.
   b. With a focused grid, cut off limits the range of focus-to-film distance.
   c. A linear grid reduces unsharpness in the image.
   d. Use of a grid may increase patient dose by a factor of 4.
   e. Grid lines in an image only occur if a stationary grid is used.

7. **In fluoroscopy with an image intensifier:**

   a. The patient entrance dose rate is typically 10–30 mGy per minute.
   b. Pulsed fluoroscopy can reduce patient entrance dose rates by up to a factor of 2.
   c. Resolution is improved when a magnified field is selected.
   d. 105 mm film images require more radiation dose than full film images.
   e. Increasing the TV camera bandwidth will improve spatial resolution.

8. **According to the Ionising Radiation (Medical Exposure) Regulations 2000 (IRMER):**

   a. Only a qualified radiologist may act as a practitioner.
   b. All referrers must undergo training.
   c. Anyone participating in the practical aspects of a medical exposure is an operator.
   d. A medical physics expert must be present for all nuclear medicine exposures.
   e. The regulations do not apply to research exposures.

9. **In radionuclide imaging with a gamma camera:**

    a. A thicker collimator (i.e. longer holes) improves resolution.
    b. Spatial resolution in the image is typically about 1 lp mm^{-1}.
    c. The purpose of the collimator is to remove scattered radiation.
    d. A thicker detecting crystal improves sensitivity.
    e. The optimum photon energy is between 100 and 300 kV.

10. **Concerning nuclear medicine procedures:**

    a. The person injecting the radionuclide into a patient is an operator, as defined in IRMER.
    b. The person injecting must hold an ARSAC certificate.
    c. It is a legal requirement to give written instructions to patients going home after a radionuclide procedure.
    d. Waiting rooms for injected patients will generally be controlled areas, as defined in IRR 1999.
    e. Radioactivity administered to patients is not covered by the Radioactive Substances Act 1993.

11. **In computed tomography (CT):**

    a. Spatial resolution is better than in film screen radiography.
    b. Contrast is improved compared with film screen radiography.
    c. A moving high attenuation object will cause a star artefact.
    d. In CT of the skull, the radiation dose at the centre of the head is similar to that at the surface.
    e. The detector is normally made from sodium iodide.

12. **In spiral CT:**

    a. Dose–length product is reduced if the pitch ratio is increased.
    b. The image can be reconstructed at any arbitrary slice position.
    c. Limitations on x-ray tube rating may result in increased noise.
    d. Image reconstruction requires interpolation of data from two complete rotations.
    e. Pitch ratio is defined as slice increment divided by section thickness.

13. **In CT:**

    a. The effective dose for a head examination is about 2 mSv.
    b. CT dose index (CTDI) is greater for a 10 mm slice width than for a 7 mm slice width.
    c. Dose–length product is measured in Gy cm^2.
    d. The effective dose for a CT abdomen is about the same as for a plain abdomen film.
    e. CTDI is measured using a thimble ionisation chamber.

14. **Deterministic effects of ionising radiation:**

    a. Are known to have resulted from interventional radiology procedures.
    b. Are an expected side effect of diagnostic nuclear medicine.
    c. Occur with a probability which is assumed to depend linearly on radiation dose.
    d. On skin will not occur at doses less than 1 Gy.
    e. Include the impairment of fertility.

15. **For the same value of dose area product given to a patient:**

    a. The effective dose will be greater if the kV is higher.
    b. Erythema is more likely if the area of skin irradiated is greater.
    c. The probability of fatal cancer is lower for a skull exposure than an abdomen exposure.
    d. For an examination of the same anatomical region, the effective dose will be independent of whether the projection is AP or PA.
    e. The entrance surface dose will decrease if the focus to skin distance is increased.

16. **Quantum mottle in a radiographic image will be increased by (assume that exposure factors are adjusted to keep the optical density of the film constant):**

    a. Using a screen with a higher conversion efficiency.
    b. Using a thicker screen.
    c. Using a higher speed film.
    d. Increasing the focus to film distance.
    e. Using an anti-scatter grid.

17. **The photoelectric effect:**

    a. Occurs only with electrons in the K shell.
    b. Can result in the production of characteristic x-rays.
    c. Occurs with free electrons.
    d. Converts all the photon's energy into kinetic energy.
    e. Is more likely if the photon's energy is only slightly greater than the electron's binding energy.

18. **In a rotating anode x-ray tube:**

    a. The anode stem is made of tungsten.
    b. The effective focal spot size depends on the anode angle.
    c. Heat is removed from the anode mainly by thermal conduction.
    d. Heat is removed more efficiently when a low tube current (mA) is used.
    e. The anode heel effect occurs in a direction parallel to the anode–cathode axis.

19. **An effective dose of 10 mSv:**

    a. Is about the average annual dose from natural radiation sources in the UK.
    b. Would give a fatal cancer risk of about 1%.
    c. Is more hazardous if it results from alpha particles than if it results from x-rays.
    d. If likely to be received during a year, would require a worker to be classified.
    e. Is the approximate dose received by a patient receiving a single AP x-ray of the abdomen.

20. **In fluoroscopy with an image intensifier:**

    a. The image on the TV monitor may have a spatial resolution as high as 5 $lp\,mm^{-1}$.
    b. The input dose rate to the image intensifier is generally less than $1\,\mu Gs^{-1}$.
    c. The input dose rate to the image intensifier will tend to increase as patient thickness increases.
    d. The input phosphor is made from zinc cadmium sulphide.
    e. Vertical resolution is determined by the number of TV scan lines.

21. **In computed radiography (CR) with a photostimulable imaging plate:**

    a. Spatial resolution of CR is significantly better than film–screen radiography.
    b. Spatial resolution in the image is determined by the size of the phosphor crystals in the image plate.
    c. A lower than optimal exposure results in a low contrast image.
    d. The system can be used with a fixed latitude.
    e. The system sensitivity (speed) can be changed after the plate has been read.

22. **When x-rays are generated at 50 kV using a tungsten target and aluminium filter:**

    a. The maximum photon energy will be 50 keV.
    b. The spectrum will have its maximum intensity at 50 keV.
    c. Characteristic radiation will not be present in the radiation emitted from the tube.
    d. X-ray output (dose per mAs) will be decreased if the filter thickness is increased.
    e. The K edge of the filter is important in shaping the x-ray spectrum.

23.   **When compression is used in mammography:**

a. It reduces the dose to the breast.
b. Its prime purpose is to immobilise the patient.
c. It reduces the proportion of scattered radiation reaching the film–screen.
d. It reduces the total volume of the breast.
e. The applied force must be less than 50 N (5 kg force).

24.   **Controlled areas (as defined by the Ionising Radiation Regulations 1999):**

a. Are not needed for mobile x-ray work.
b. Are not needed if the x-ray room has a protective screen.
c. Normally extend beyond the confines of the x-ray room.
d. Are needed for rooms where patients are injected with a radionuclide.
e. Must have restrictions on who may enter them.

25.   **Quality assurance in diagnostic x-ray work:**

a. Is required by the Ionising Radiation Regulations 1999.
b. Is required by Ionising Radiation (Medical Exposure) Regulations 2000.
c. Is the responsibility of the Radiation Protection Adviser.
d. Need cover only x-ray and associated equipment.
e. Requires all equipment tests to be done at least yearly.

1. **Answers**

   a. **True** – the K shell electrons are closer to the nucleus and are subject to a greater attractive force.
   b. **True** – the binding energies of electrons are fixed values.
   c. **False** – the atomic number defines which element an atom is, and corresponds to the number of protons in the nucleus.
   d. **False** – the outer electron shell defines the diameter of an atom. This has a diameter tens of thousands of times the diameter of the nucleus.
   e. **False** – while there are normally more neutrons than protons in heavy nuclei, it is common to find equal numbers, or an excess of protons in light nuclei. For example, hydrogen (1p, 0n), helium (2p, 2n), carbon-12 (6p, 6n).

2. **Answers**

   a. **True** – a neutron is converted to a proton and an electron (the beta particle). The atomic number is increased by 1.
   b. **True** – a nucleus that emits a positron does so by converting a proton to a neutron, to conserve electric charge. The fact that it needed to reduce the number of protons indicates that there was initially an excess of protons.
   c. **False** – Molybdenum-99 decays to technetium-99m. Technetium cannot then decay back to molybdenum. Technetium-99m decays to technetium-99, which then decays to stable ruthenium-99.
   d. **True** – like electrons in their shells, the particles in a nucleus have binding energies. A gamma ray has an energy corresponding to the difference between two energy levels in a nucleus. Although a nuclide may emit several gamma rays of different energies, the spectrum is not continuous.
   e. **False** – although beta decay involves a fixed energy change within the nucleus, the energy is shared between the beta particle and a neutrino. This means that the beta particle can have any energy up to a fixed maximum. The maximum represents the situation where the electron takes all the available energy.

3. **Answers**

a. **True** – if the photon has less energy than the binding energy, the electron will not be ejected from its shell. With only slightly more than the binding energy, the photon will be absorbed, resulting in a photoelectric interaction. With much more than the binding energy, the photon will interact with the electron as if the electron were free.

b. **False** – a high energy photon loses much more of its energy than a low energy photon.

c. **False** – although the photon can be deflected backwards, the electron cannot be deflected by more than 90° to the initial direction of the photon. If the electron were deflected through more than 90°, it would be moving 'backwards'. In order to conserve momentum, the photon's momentum in the 'forward' direction would have to increase. Both the photon and electron would have gained kinetic energy, which would violate the principle of conservation of energy.

d. **False** – scatter results in photons being deflected from their original path. Since diagnostic imaging depends on knowing the path of a photon from its point of origin to a point in the image, Compton scatter will tend to degrade the image.

e. **False** – over the range of photon energies used in diagnostic x-ray imaging, the probability of Compton scatter remains about the same. At higher energies the probability decreases slowly. The probability of photoelectric interactions decreases much more rapidly as photon energy increases, so that Compton scatter becomes a much greater proportion of the total number of events.

4. **Answers**

a. **False** – the maximum photon energy depends on the energy of the electrons striking the target. The maximum electron energy will depend upon the maximum potential applied across the tube. This is the same for both types of generator.

b. **True** – (and c and d) with a high frequency generator, the tube potential will be close to its peak value throughout the exposure, whereas in a single phase set, the potential will vary between zero and the peak kV. So for most of the time, the high frequency set is operating at a greater tube potential than the single phase set, resulting in higher mean photon energy, a greater half value thickness and greater x-ray output.

c. **True** – see b.

d. **True** – see b.

e. **False** – the voltage waveform makes no difference, in practice, to the heel effect. Since the higher energy photons are more penetrating, the heel effect would, if anything, be less pronounced at the higher mean photon energies produced by a high frequency generator.

5. **Answers**

   a. **True** – it is common to have both molybdenum and rhodium or tungsten targets.
   b. **False** – typical tube voltages are 25 kV to 32 kV.
   c. **False** – the axial ray is the central ray of the x-ray beam. The tube is usually angled so that the axial ray is at the chest wall edge of the field. This is to make use of the anode heel effect so as to produce a more uniform exposure of the film.
   d. **False** – it is essential for the anode to rotate, to allow enough x-rays to be produced from a small focal spot, within the heat rating.
   e. **False** – focal spot sizes need to be smaller than this to enable fine structures to be resolved in the image. Typically the size is 0.3 mm for normal views, and 0.1 mm for magnified views.

6. **Answers**

   a. **True** – far from the centre of the x-ray field, the photons are travelling at a greater angle to the normal, so a greater number are cut off by a parallel grid.
   b. **True** – the strips making up the grid are set at an angle that matches the angle of travel of the x-rays from the focus. This matching is only perfect at a certain focus-to-film distance, and only within a range close to the ideal FFD will the degree of cut off remain within acceptable limits.
   c. **False** – a grid improves contrast rather than unsharpness.
   d. **True** – grids always increase patient dose because they absorb useful radiation, requiring greater exposures. The increase can be as high as a factor of 4.
   e. **False** – grid lines may be seen with a moving grid if it has to change direction during the exposure. Grid lines may also be seen if the grid moves by a distance equal to a whole number of grid spacings, between each peak of the voltage waveform.

7. **Answers**

   a. **True** – for slim patients and large field sizes, dose rates below 10 mGy per minute should be achievable, but the range quoted in the question is typical.
   b. **True** – although a higher tube current is used, x-ray production occurs for only a small fraction of the time, so that doses are lower by using a lower acquired frame rate. Greater reductions than this are possible, at the expense of some jerkiness in moving images.
   c. **True** – the image details are magnified, allowing better resolution of finer detail.
   d. **False** – they require about 1 μGy per image (detector dose) compared with about 10 μGy for full film images.
   e. **True** – at the expense of increased noise.

8. **Answers**

   a. **False** – a practitioner can be a health professional entitled to act in this capacity by the employer's procedures.
   b. **False** – referrers need to be made aware of the employer's referral procedures, but they do not need to be trained.
   c. **True** – as stated in the 'guide to good practice' which accompanies the regulations.
   d. **False** – an expert must be available for diagnostic procedures.
   e. **False** – they apply to all medical exposures of people.

9. **Answers**

   a. **True** – it reduces the range of angles from which photons can reach the detector, so limiting the uncertainty in determining their point of origin.
   b. **False** – resolution is normally no better than 5 mm.
   c. **False** – the collimator restricts the radiation entering the detector to photons travelling in the direction of the collimator holes. Scattered radiation is discriminated by the pulse height measurement in the camera.
   d. **True** – it does this by detecting a greater proportion of the photons.
   e. **True** – this energy range represents a compromise between detection efficiency and absorption of photons within the patient.

10. **Answers**

   a. **True** – injection of the radionuclide is a practical aspect of the exposure.
   b. **False** – the person justifying the exposure (the practitioner) must hold a certificate, but the person injecting need not.
   c. **False** – it is a requirement to have a procedure that states when and how instructions must be given. The procedure might not require instructions in all cases.
   d. **True** – the dose rate from several injected patients will usually be great enough to require a controlled area.
   e. **False** – keeping the radioactive material requires registration under the Act. Disposal from hospital premises, by a patient going to the lavatory, requires a disposal authorisation.

11. **Answers**

   a. False – resolution is generally poorer, about 1 lp mm^{-1}, compared with 5–10 lp mm^{-1} in film radiography.
   b. True – it is at least 10 times better because there are no overlying structures in the image, and windowing allows small contrast levels to be made visible.
   c. False – a moving object will cause a streak artefact. Its movement will cause it to appear in different scan lines as the scan progresses. A star artefact is caused by a stationary high attenuation (usually metallic) object, which has a Hounsfield number so great that the image reconstruction algorithm is unable to allocate it to a single pixel.
   d. False – it is 50% of the surface dose.
   e. False – detectors used include solid-state detectors and xenon-filled ionisation chambers. Sodium iodide is used in gamma cameras.

12. **Answers**

   a. True – increasing the pitch means that the same volume is scanned in fewer revolutions. The same dose per revolution is used, so the dose–length product is smaller.
   b. True – image reconstruction requires interpolation between the data for adjacent rotations. Since rotation is continuous, the reconstruction can be referred to an arbitrary position in a rotation, allowing any slice within the scanned volume to be reconstructed.
   c. True – in helical scans, the tube is producing x-rays continuously, and there is less time for cooling. The increased heat loading on the tube limits the maximum tube current, so reducing the maximum dose rate. This will reduce the number of photons producing each pixel.
   d. False – in 180° interpolation, the data from two half rotations are used, i.e. one complete rotation.
   e. True – sometimes this is referred to simply as pitch.

13. **Answers**

   a. True.
   b. False – the dose integrated over 100 mm (or 150 mm using some definitions of CTDI) will vary in proportion to slice width. However, this value is divided by the slice width to give CTDI, so that CTDI remains constant. The CTDI would be greater for the 7 mm slice if the mAs per rotation were increased to reduce noise.
   c. False – the correct unit is Gy cm or mGy cm.
   d. False – the CT will be about 7 mSv, compared with about 1 mSv for the plain film.
   e. False – a pencil ionisation chamber is used, to achieve a measurement over the required length.

14. **Answers**

   a. **True** – although rare, some deterministic skin effects have occurred following interventional procedures.
   b. **False** – deterministic effects do not occur in properly conducted examinations.
   c. **False** – deterministic effects occur over a fairly well defined range of doses – hence the term 'deterministic'. Since there is a range of dose below a threshold, where the probability is zero, the variation cannot be linear.
   d. **True** – the threshold dose is around 2 Gy.
   e. **True** – the threshold dose is between 0.2 and 2 Gy, depending on age, sex, dose fractionation and whether temporary or permanent impairment is considered.

15. **Answers**

   a. **True** – usually increasing the kV reduces patient dose, because the radiation is more penetrating – but this relies on being able to reduce the mAs to take advantage of this. In this question, the dose area product remains constant, so the increase in kV results in greater doses to the tissues below the skin surface. This results in a greater effective dose.
   b. **False** – the dose area product is dose multiplied by the area. If the area is greater, then the dose required to get the same dose area product is smaller, and the smaller dose is less likely to be above the erythema threshold.
   c. **True** – the tissues thought to be most sensitive to cancer induction are in the abdomen. The lower probability of cancer from a skull x-ray will be reflected in the lower effective dose for the same dose area product.
   d. **False** – the effective dose will depend upon the location of those tissues with significant weighting factors. The projection chosen affects the doses to such tissues significantly. An example is the dose to the breasts in chest radiography, which is higher for an AP than a PA chest radiograph.
   e. **True** – if the focus–skin distance is increased, the field size will increase. The dose required to achieve the same dose area product will be smaller.

16. **Answers**

   a. **True** – the screen produces more light per x-ray photon, so fewer x-ray photons are needed.
   b. **False** – the screen will stop a greater proportion of the photons, so although fewer are incident on the screen, the same number are used to form the image.
   c. **True** – less light is needed to produce the image on the film, so fewer x-ray photons are required to produce the same optical density.
   d. **False** – the same number of photons are used to produce the image.
   e. **False** – the grid improves contrast in the image. There will be no difference in the amount of mottle as exposure will have been adjusted.

17. **Answers**

   a. **False** – it can occur with any shell, though the photon energy likely to produce the effect in the outer shell electron may be below that used in diagnostic radiology.
   b. **True** – when the vacancy caused by the liberated photoelectron is filled, a characteristic photon is emitted.
   c. **False** – Compton scatter occurs with free electrons.
   d. **False** – part of the photon's energy is used to overcome the electron's binding energy. The rest is given to the electron as kinetic energy.
   e. **True** – resonance effects mean that photoelectric interactions are favoured when the photon energy only marginally exceeds the electron's binding energy.

18. **Answers**

   a. **False** – it is made of molybdenum, to reduce heat conduction to the bearings.
   b. **True** – at shallower angles (as viewed from the x-ray tube window), the focal spot is foreshortened.
   c. **False** – radiation is the prime heat removal mechanism.
   d. **False** – heat loss by radiation is proportional to the fourth power of the absolute temperature. A high tube current results in faster heat deposition in the target, and a higher temperature.
   e. **True** – in this direction, the x-ray output varies because of differential absorption of x-rays in the target resulting from angulation of the target.

19. **Answers**

   a. **False** – the mean is about 2.2 mSv.
   b. **False** – the International Committee of Radiation Protection quotes a risk of about 1 in 20 000 per mSv of a fatal cancer. So for 10 mSv, the risk is about 1 in 2000, or 0.05%.
   c. **False** – this would be true for absorbed dose, but effective dose incorporates a radiation weighting factor to account for the increased risk associated with exposure to alpha particles.
   d. **True** – employees must be classified if they are likely to exceed 6 mSv in a year.
   e. **False** – a normal size patient should only receive 1 mSv or less from an abdominal x-ray.

20. **Answers**

   a. **False** – even with zoom field sizes, the achievable resolution is only about 3.5 lp mm^{-1}.
   b. **True** – this is not a limit, but most systems should be capable of producing a satisfactory image using dose rates lower than this.
   c. **False** – the automatic brightness control will keep the image intensifier input dose rate approximately constant, though the patient dose rate will increase. For very large patients, the input dose rate will decrease, as the set will reach its exposure rate limit.
   d. **False** – sodium activated caesium iodide is used.
   e. **True** – vertical refers to the direction from the top to bottom of the monitor. To resolve a line pair requires two scan lines, so the more lines that form the image, the greater the number of line pairs that can be resolved.

21. **Answers**

   a. **False** – the spatial resolution is similar, high-resolution CR having a maximum spatial resolution of 10 lp mm^{-1}.
   b. **False** – the main limit on spatial resolution is the diameter of the laser scanning spot and scattering of the laser light in the image plate.
   c. **False** – the reader will increase its sensitivity if a lower exposure is used, producing the same displayed contrast. However the smaller number of photons per pixel will make the image noisier.
   d. **True** – this can be selected by the operator.
   e. **False** – once the plate has been read, the pixel values are fixed. Although the image can be windowed, the sensitivity cannot be changed.

22. **Answers**

a. **True** – this is the maximum energy of the electrons.
b. **False** – the peak intensity will occur at an energy about one third of the peak energy.
c. **True** – the electrons do not have enough energy to produce K x-rays. Although L x-rays will be produced, they will be insufficiently penetrating to escape the tube.
d. **True** – the filter absorbs a proportion of the x-rays, so increasing its thickness will reduce the number of x-ray photons emerging from the tube.
e. **False** – the K edge of aluminium is 1.6 keV. The K edge has no effect on the shape of the spectrum.

23. **Answers**

a. **True** – there is a smaller thickness of tissue for the x-ray beam to penetrate, so a smaller entrance dose can be used.
b. **False** – this isn't its prime purpose, though it is a useful outcome!
c. **True** – the lower exposure means that fewer scattering events occur. Although a smaller proportion are absorbed within the compressed breast (because it is thinner), the overall effect is of fewer scattered photons compared with primary photons reaching each part of the image.
d. **False** – compression just squashes the breast into a different shape. It does not reduce the volume.
e. **False** – compression forces up to 200 N are permitted.

24. **Answers**

a. **False** – you still need a controlled area, though it is not necessary to physically demarcate it.
b. **False** – you still need a controlled area. Some hospitals choose to include the area protected by the screen as part of the controlled area.
c. **False** – good practice is to design an x-ray room so that dose rates outside are low enough not to need to be controlled or supervised.
d. **False** – the need for a controlled area depends on the dose rate and the need for precautions. It may be possible to avoid designating the area.
e. **True** – only classified employees, and those entering in accordance with written arrangements, may enter controlled areas.

25.   **Answers**

   a. **True** – relating to quality assurance of equipment.
   b. **True** – relating to quality assurance of procedures.
   c. **False** – it is the responsibility of the employer, whichever of the two sets of regulations are considered.
   d. **False** – it needs to cover procedures as well.
   e. **False** – the regulations specify tests 'at appropriate intervals'. For some tests it is appropriate to perform them less than once per year.